Responder Chem-Bio Handbook

A Practical Manual for First Responders

Version 1.5

Possible chemical or biological attacks contain a multitude of variables which are impossible to predict. This book aims to provide you with general information that can be applied to most situations but is by no means the final word on what actions you should take. The handbook is meant to be a supplement to actual training and is not to be used as the sole guide for diagnosis and treatment. No book is a substitute for hands-on training from expert instructors. Medical treatment in any particular case should always be based upon proper medical evaluation and training and not on the contents of this handbook.

ISBN 0-9665437-0-X

Voice: (703) 370-2962   Fax: (703) 370-1571
Email: publishing@tempestco.com
Web: www.tempestco.com/publishing
PO Box 22572, Alexandria, VA 22304-9257 USA

SECTION A

Actions

A-1 - Scene Assessment and Control

A-2 - Indicators of Chem-Bio Attack

A-3 - Personal Protective Equipment

A-4 - Protective Levels - PPE

A-1 - Scene Assessment and Control

The most important actions for a first responder when confronting a WMD Chemical/Biological incident are the initial scene assessment and gaining control of the situation as it evolves. These pre-planed actions will mean the difference between life and death for yourself and the public for whom you are responsible.

While responding to the scene, begin mentally performing an initial assessment of the current situation composed of:
- Incident Assessment
- Establishing a manageable perimeter.
- Establish control zones and areas.
- Public protection considerations.
- Evacuation vs. In-place sheltering
- Scene security
- Tactical considerations

I. INITIAL ASSESSMENT
A. Enroute
- Remember to expect the unexpected!
- Assess nature and description of call.
- If necessary, ask for additional units to be activated and await further instructions.
- Consider best possible access to scene.
- If unfamiliar with the area/location ask for assistance and best possible route starting at least two blocks from the incident.
- If an explosive device was involved, access to the scene may be limited due to debris.
- Determine wind direction.
- No matter what the incident description, always suspect an airborne hazard is present and approach the scene from upwind.
- Consider what equipment will be needed to provide protection for you and your crew (turnout gear, SCBA, Level-A HazMat suit).
- Anticipate the possibility of multiple

hazards, natural and man-made, present at the scene.
• Could there be secondary devices present on scene?
• Could there be terrorists still on the scene?
• Consider that terrorists could be among the injured or close by the scene.

B. Upon Arrival
• Isolate hazard area and control exodus of panicked and contaminated people.
• Identify and evaluate dangers.
• Estimate perimeter boundaries
• Best to over-estimate perimeters.
• Outer perimeter - most distant boundary.
• Inner perimeter - isolates known hazards within outer perimeter.
• Perimeter entry and exit points
• Assess available personal protective equipment (PPE).

C. Incident Assessment

• This is a continual process that will help you to determine type/degree of hazard you are confronting.
• What is the present situation?
• What is causing the problem?
• What is the life safety risk?
• What is the stability of the incident?
• What are current weather conditions (sun, rain, wind)?

D. Establish control zones and areas

• Hot zone – restricted access
• Warm zone
• Cold zone – staging area
• Decontamination area
• Triage and treatment area

E. Public Protection

• Evacuation of the public from danger determined by:
  • Degree or severity of dangers.
  • Number of individuals or affected population.
  • Available resources to assist

evacuation.
- Means to notify public, i.e., media, public address system
- Safe route and refuge area
- Evacuees with special needs, i.e. hearing/sight impaired, wheelchairs
- Safer to remain in place vs. evacuate
- Combination of both evacuation and remaining in place

F. Scene Security
- Initial scene security will be chaotic but must be accomplished.
- *Units must enforce perimeter continuity.*
- *Not everyone can be involved in the actual incident.*
- Incident Commander responsible for all entry and exit routes from site.
- Early in the incident, security will be a combination of police and fire personnel.
- Transition scene security to law enforcement totally as incident stabilizes.
- Military units may be required – dependent on magnitude of incident.

G. Tactical Considerations

- Always approach scene with caution utilizing PPE when warranted.
- Potential for secondary incident.
- Be alert for signs of danger.
- Casualties for no apparent reason.
- Signs and symptoms of chemical exposure being exhibited.
- Signs of criminal activity, i.e., weapons or suspected explosive device.
- Pre-incident threat, i.e., written or verbal.
- Proper staging of vehicles.
- Avoid visible vapor, mist and unknown liquid.
- Assign one responder as an observer.
- Be alert for criminal activity.
- Plan escape routes and refuge area.
- Prepare for emergency decontamination during all phases of incident.

II. Scene Management
A. Role of Incident Commander during a CB Incident

- Establish command
- Hazard and risk assessment
- Notifications to other responders and local government.
- Site safety
- Ensure responder protection levels.
- Public protection
- Develop and implement integrated incident action plans.
- Control hazards
- Request specialized resources.
- Logistical support
- Information control
- Incident termination
- Document and evaluate total response to improve future response.

Actions For IC to Follow
• Establish goals and objectives for the overall response.

Resources
• What is needed?
• Where can you get it?
• How long will it take to arrive?
• What specialized crews or training do you require?
• What agencies should be involved in the response?

Plan and Structure
• Determine and assign responsibilities and tasks!
• Establish a Chain of Command (COC).
• Plan and define any coordination issues relative to response.

Take Action
• Mobilize your resources.
• Establish a Command Post (CP).
• Establish staging and receiving areas.
• Isolate the area.

- Treat and rescue victims.
- Establish inner and outer working zones.
- Establish access routes.
- Issue warnings.
- Initiate further evacuation if required.
- Establish liaisons with media and other agencies.

Notes:

CHEMICAL ATTACK INDICATORS:
The following section contains indicators to
help identify whether a chemical attack has
occurred.

Indicator - Description
Dead animals/birds and fish - Not just the
occasional road kill, but numerous dead
animals (domestic and wild, small or large
dead) in the same area.

Lack of insect life - If normal insect activity
is missing, check the surrounding area
(ground/water surface/shoreline) for dead
insects. If near the water, check the area for
dead fish and aquatic birds.

Blisters/rashes - Numerous individuals
experiencing unexplained water-like blisters,
wheal (like bee-stings), and/or rashes.

Mass Casualties - Numerous individuals
exhibiting unexplained serious health

problems ranging from nausea and vomiting, difficulty breathing, or unexplained unconsciousness.

Patterns of Casualties - Victims are distributed in a pattern associated with a specific agent dispersal (line source/point).

Illness associated with enclosed areas vs. open areas - A definite pattern of victims which can be associated to a release. Indoors vs. outdoors.

Unusual liquid droplets or puddles - Numerous surfaces in the surrounding area exhibit oily droplets/film or puddles. Or numerous water surfaces have an oily film present (no rain).

Areas which look different in visual appearance - Not just a patch of dead weeds, but surrounding plant life, trees, and lawns are dead, discolored or appear withered (no current drought).

Unexplained odors -
Odors in the area can be:
- Bitter Almonds/peach kernels
- Newly mown hay or green grass

Low-lying clouds - Low-lying clouds/fog like conditions which is contrary to the current weather conditions. (sunny and foggy)

Unusual objects or debris in area - Visual recognition of some sort of dissemination device. Unexploded or released material in the area. Items which contain liquid on site or remain in the area.

Notes:

BIOLOGICAL ATTACK INDICATORS:

The following section contains indicators to help identify whether a biological attack has occurred.

Indicators - Description

An unusual number of sick or dead people and animals within an area or location. - Any number of symptoms can be present in a suspected biological attack. As a first responder you should consider assessing (polling) the local area hospitals to see if additional casualties with similar symptoms have been observed.

Casualties can present in minutes, hours, days and even weeks after an incident has occurred.

The time required before symptoms are observed in a biological attack is dependent upon the actual agent used.

Abandoned spray devices - These devices have no odor or identifiable marks.

Unscheduled and unusual spraying - This can usually be the first indication that an attack of some kind has occurred within a specific area or location.

Patterns of Casualties - Victims which are distributed in such a pattern which is associated with a specific dispersal method (food poisoning).

Notes:

Introduction:
Personal protective equipment for use against CB agents is designed to consist of methods which prevent toxic or infectious materials from contacting the body, internally or externally. The methods described below will provide the first responder with sufficient levels of protection in a suspected or known CB event. However, the protection levels required during an event may vary depending upon the specific agent encountered, the conditions under which the protective clothing and devices (respirators) are worn and the activities (rescue, decon, recovery/mitigation) which the individual is engaged in.

Levels of Protection:
Personal protective equipment is divided into four categories based on the degree of protection afforded the rescuer.

Equipment and Recommended Uses: LEVEL-A

A Level-A suit provides the greatest level of skin, respiratory and eye protection to the rescuer.

A Level-A suit is comprised of:

- Pressure-demand, full face-piece, SCBA.
- Vapor protection suit (totally encapsulating) airtight suit, consisting of the following criteria:
    - Covers the full torso, head, arms and legs.
    - Includes boots and gloves, which may be part of the suit or attached.
    - Completely encloses the user and his or her SCBA, gloves and boots.
    - Two-way radio equipment enclosed within the suit.

Recommended Uses:

A Level-A suit should be used under any of the following conditions:

- When a material, (CW or other) requires the highest level of protection for skin, eyes, and the respiratory system based on either the measured (or potential) high concentration of atmospheric vapors, gases, or particles.

• When the environment has a high risk of splash potential, immersion, or exposure to unexpected vapors, gases, or particles.

• When substances with a high degree of hazard to the skin are known or suspected to be present and skin contact is possible.

• When operations need to be conducted in a confined, poorly ventilated area, and/or required level of equipment has yet to be determined.

LEVEL-B

A Level-B suit provides the rescuer with the highest level of respiratory protection when necessary and a lesser level of skin protection.

A Level-B suit is comprised of:

• Pressure-demand, full face-piece, SCBA or pressure-demand air line

respirator with escape SCBA.
- Hooded chemical-resistant clothing consisting of the following:
  - Coveralls
  - Gloves inner and outer
  - Boots
  - Hard-hat
  - Face Shield (optional)
  - Two-Way radios

Recommended Uses:

A Level-B suit is recommended when:
- The type and atmospheric concentration of a substance has been identified and requires a high level of respiratory protection, but less skin protection.
- The atmosphere contains less then 19.5% oxygen.
- The presence of identified vapors or gases is indicated by detection methods, and the vapor or gases are known not to contain high levels of chemicals harmful to the skin or capable of being absorbed through intact skin.
- The presence of liquids or particles is

indicated, but they are known not to contain high levels of chemicals harmful to skin or capable of being absorbed through intact skin.

LEVEL-C

A Level-C suit provides the rescuer with a level of protection which is adequate when the concentration(s) and type(s) of airborne substance(s) are known and the criteria for using air-purifying respirators are met.
A Level-C suit is comprised of:

- Full-face shield or half mask
- Air purifying respirator, or SCBA
- Hooded chemical-resistant clothing consisting of the following:
    - Coveralls
    - Gloves inner and outer
    - Boots
    - Hard-hat
    - Face Shield (optional)
    - Two-Way radios

Recommended Uses:

A Level-C suit is recommended when:

  • The levels of contaminate, liquid splashes or other direct contact will not adversely affect or be absorbed through any exposed skin.

  • The types of chemicals have been identified, concentrations have been measured, and an air-purifying respirator is available that can remove contaminates.

  • The atmosphere contains at least 19.5% oxygen.

LEVEL-D

A Level-D suit is a work uniform which affords a rescuer with minimal protection.

Recommended Uses:

A Level-D suit is recommended when:

  • The atmosphere contains no known hazards.

  • Work functions preclude splashes, immersion, or the potential for unexpected inhalation of any chemicals.

** Protection Level C and D are not applicable to the initial entry and response at the scene of a CW attack. In most cases responders will not know the type and concentration of the agent involved.

**Chemical Protective Clothing (CPC) is made from special materials and designed to prevent the contact of chemicals with the body.

**Air Purifying Respirators are devices, which are worn to filter particles and contaminants from the air. They are often the only levels of protection required when a biological agent is suspected. They are specifically designed to be worn in atmospheres where the type and quantity of contaminates are known and sufficient oxygen is known to be present. They are simple, cheap, and offer specific protection to the user.

A-4 - Protective Levels - PPE

Chemical Agent	Vapor	Liquid
VX	Level A	Level A, B, C*
Sarin (GB)	Level A	Level A, B, C*
Tabun (GA)	Level A	Level A, B, C*
Soman (GD)	Level A	Level A, B, C*
Distilled Mustard (HD)	Level A	Level A, B, C*
Nitrogen Mustard (HN)	Level A	Level A, B, C*
Sulfur Mustard (H)	Level A	Level A, B, C*
Phosgene Oxime (CX)	Level A	Level A, B, C*
Lewisite (L)	Level A	Level A, B, C*
Phenyldichloroarsine (PD)	Level A	Level A, B, C*
Ethyldichloroarsine (ED)	Level A	Level A, B, C*
Phosgene (CG)	Level A	Level B, C*
Chlorine (CL)	Level B, C	Level B, C*

Chemical Agent	Vapor	Liquid
Hydrogen Cyanide (AC)	Level A	Level B, C*
Cyanogen Chloride (CK)	Level B, C	Level B, C*
Adamsite	Level B, C	Level B, C*

Level-C protection level is dependent on the operational assignment. See recommended guidelines in previous section regarding proper use of Level-C PPE.

Notes:

<u>Biological Agents</u>

B-1 - Introduction

B-2 - Bacteria

B-3 - Toxins

B-4 - Viruses

Biological warfare is the intentional use of organisms or chemicals of biological origin to cause death and disease among personnel, animals, and plants, or to deteriorate material.

When considering biological attacks from the perspective of a first responder, it is important to note that, with the exception of some of the toxins, any physical manifestations of an attack are likely to be delayed. Therefore, response to a biological attack is largely an investigative matter researched by epidemiologists through manifested symptomology. This chapter will review some of the characteristics of biological agents, types of potential biological agents, detection, attack indicators, diagnosis, therapy, contamination issues, and protective measures. Although there are innumerable potential biological agents, only a few are regarded as being rational choices for aggressors. The agents profiled in this chapter are those that have either been weaponized by nations with weapons programs and/or have been used or sought by terrorists.

Biological agents are governed by intrinsic features which influence their utility as weapons. Among these features are:
- Infectivity
- Virulence
- Toxicity
- Pathogenicity
- Incubation period
- Transmissibility
- Lethality
- Stability

Infectivity

The infectivity of an agent is a measure of the relative ease with which microorganisms establish themselves in a host species. Thus, the more infective an agent is, the fewer organisms required to cause disease.

Virulence

The virulence of an agent reflects the relative severity of disease produced by that agent.

Toxicity

The toxicity of an agent reflects the relative severity of illness or incapacitation produced by a toxin.

Pathogenicity

This reflects the capability of an infectious agent to cause disease in a susceptible host.

Incubation Period

The time between exposure and the appearance of symptoms. Microorganisms require time to multiply (replicate) within a host before they reach a sufficient number to produce disease. The duration of the incubation period is governed by many variables, including: the initial dose; virulence; route of entry; rate of replication; and a host of immunological factors.

Transmissibility
The relative ease with which an agent is passed from person-to-person.

Lethality
Lethality reflects the relative ease with which an agent causes death in a susceptible population.

Stability
A quantitative measure of stability is an agent's decay rate. This a measure of an agent's susceptibility to various environmental factors such as, temperature, relative humidity, atmospheric pollution, and sunlight.

Additional Factors
Additional factors which may influence the suitability of a microorganism or toxin as a biological weapon include: ease of production; stability when stored or transported; and ease of dissemination.

Types of Potential Biological Agents:

Bacteria

Bacteria are small free-living organisms, most of which may be grown on solid or liquid culture media. The organisms have a structure consisting of nuclear material, cytoplasm, and cell membrane. They reproduce by simple division. The diseases they produce often respond to specific therapy with antibiotics.

Viruses

Viruses are organisms which require living cells in which to replicate. They are therefore intimately dependent upon the cells of the host which they infect. They produce diseases which generally do not respond to antibiotics but which may be responsive to antiviral compounds, of which there are few available, and those that are available are of limited use.

Rickettsiae

Rickettsiae are microorganisms which have characteristics common to both bacteria and viruses. Like bacteria, they possess metabolic enzymes and cell membranes, utilize oxygen, and are susceptible to broad-spectrum antibiotics. They resemble viruses in that they grow only within living cells.

Chlamydia

Chlamydia are obligatory intracellular parasites incapable of generating their own energy source. Like bacteria, they are responsive to broad-spectrum antibiotics. Like viruses, they require living cells for multiplication.

Fungi

Fungi are distinct from plants, animals, and bacteria. Although they appear to grow like plants, they do not photosynthesize and usually live on live or dead plant or animal matter and with only a few exceptions are aerobic (needing oxygen for growth). They include microscopic yeasts and large mushrooms and are spread by spores that can be an operationally effective method for dispersing agents. Infections are resistant to antibacterial antibiotics and can be difficult and dangerous to treat.

Toxins
Toxins are poisonous substances produced and derived from living plants, animals, or microorganisms; some toxins may also be produced or altered by chemical means. Toxins may be countered by specific antisera and selected pharmacologic agents.

Collectively, biological agents other than toxins are also known as live agents. Live agents are living organisms. Unique to many of these agents is the ability to multiply in the body over time and actually increase their effect. For some agents, only a few organisms are needed to cause infection. Once a casualty is infected, agents require time to multiply enough to overcome the body's defenses. This incubation period may vary from hours to days or weeks depending on the type of organism.

Live agents have life cycles in which to grow, reproduce, age, and die. These agents usually require protection and nutrition supplied by another living organism (the host) to survive and grow. Weathering (wind, rain, and sunlight) rapidly reduces their numbers. Some bacterial agents produce spores that can form protective coats and survive longer. However, the hazard from most live agents may only last for one day.

Detection

Live agents are not detectable by any of the five physical senses; usually the first indication of a biological attack is the initial observed casualty. Human beings are a sensitive, and in some cases the only, biodetector. Early clinical findings may be nonspecific or atypical of the natural disease. Medical personnel may be unable to differentiate natural disease from BW attacks. Considerable time may elapse following a BW attack before the extent of the exposure is appreciated.

Attack Indicators

Biological attacks are likely to be covert, making detection reliant on symptomology. Even if symptoms are expressed, epidemiologic research must be employed to determine whether the symptoms are typical of a background endemic disease or a unique event. Mixed infections or intoxications may occur and complicate or delay diagnosis. A large number of casualties may occur during a short period of time with anywhere from a few patients with flu-like symptoms to a full mass casualty event. Other points to note for recognition include:
  • A disease pattern with characteristics that differ from those of a naturally-occurring epidemic
  • Disease incidence increasing within a period of a few hours or days
  • A compressed, epidemic curve
  • A steady and increasing stream of

patients arriving at health care facilities.
• An illness type highly unusual for the geographic area.
• An unusually high prevalence of respiratory involvement in diseases that typically causes a non-pulmonary syndrome.
• Casualty distribution aligned with wind direction.
• Lower attack rates among those working indoors, especially in areas with filtered air or closed ventilation systems, than in those exposed outdoors.
• Increased numbers of sick or dead animals, often of different species.
• Witness to an attack, or discovery of an appropriate delivery system.
• Large numbers of rapidly fatal cases, with few recognizable signs and symptoms, resulting from exposure to multiple lethal doses near the dissemination source.

Diagnosis

Accurate reporting of clinical findings may be critical in alerting other responders to both the possibility and nature of a BW attack. Unfortunately, attempts to reach an accurate diagnosis on clinical grounds alone may not be possible. Specialized diagnostic kits may provide field identification capabilities. However, these kits are in limited availability and are prohibitively expensive for responders. Any provisional identification will require specialized laboratory analysis to establish definitive diagnosis.

Antibiotic Therapy

Antibiotics must be given to all BW casualties, even without a firm diagnosis. Most bacterial, chlamydial, and rickettsial diseases respond to antibiotics. The choice of drug depends on the clinical circumstances, but one broad-spectrum antibiotic should be administered in full therapeutic doses, parenterally if possible, and preferably intravenously, and commenced at the earliest possible level of medical care.

Decontamination (also see Section D):
Primary Contamination

Dermal exposure from a suspected BW attack should be managed by decontamination at the earliest opportunity. In the absence of agent-specific guidance, exposed areas should be cleansed using an appropriately diluted sodium hypochlorite solution (0.5%) or copious quantities of plain soap and water. This should follow any needed use of decontaminants for chemical agents but should be prompt. Potentially contaminated clothing should be removed as soon as is practical by protected personnel (that is, in full PPE) in an area away from non-contaminated patients. Following decontamination, the casualty should be protected from further exposure.

Secondary Contamination

Secondary contamination of medical personnel from clothing or equipment of exposed casualties may be important. This is particularly worrisome from casualties recently exposed near the dissemination source where high levels of contamination may occur. Since it will be difficult to distinguish those casualties exposed near the source from those contaminated some distance away, proper physical protection of health care providers or other persons handling exposed personnel should be maintained until decontamination is complete.

Protection of First Responder
Following decontamination, patients are cared for using standard techniques including universal infectious disease precautions (barrier nursing). Protection of first responders is offered through use of impermeable surgical gowns/oral-nasal masks/face shields or goggles/surgical gloves and observance of universal (body fluid) precautions/barrier nursing techniques. However, it should be noted that not all biological agents pose a hazard for secondary transmission.

In the context of biological agent casualties, adherence to principles of patient isolation is essential to preventing cross-infection with transmissible agents. Separation of non-affected individuals from contaminated victims of biological agent attack (cohorting; reverse quarantine) and implementation of barrier nursing procedures should be initiated as soon as practical after a BW incident.

Notes:

Diagnostic Table

The following data is an adapted version of the data presented in the US Department of the Army publication, *Handbook on the Medical Aspects of NBC Defensive Operations - FM 8-9; Part II - Biological, Annex D - Table II, An Approach to Potential BW Agents by Clinical Finding or Syndrome, 1 February 1996.*

Potential Causes - These lists are not comprehensive. For illustrative purposes only, not to be used as a clinical guide.

Syndrome	General Characteristics	Potential Causes
Diarrhea-dysentery	Typically with fever	Shigella
Diarrhea-watery	With or without fever	Cholera Ebola/Marburg Lassa fever Staphylococcus enterotoxin B
Encephalitis/ encephalopathy	With or without fever	Argentine hemorrhagic fever Bolivian hemorrhagic fever Eastern equine encephalitis Lassa fever Plague Psittacosis Rift Valley fever (infrequent) Russian spring-summer encephalitis Venezuelan equine encephalitis Western equine encephalitis

Syndrome	General Characteristics	Potential Causes
Fever		Any (Toxins less likely)
Flaccid paralysis	Sensory paresthesias, flaccid weakness, cranial nerve abnormalities	Botulinum toxins Saxitoxin Tetradotoxin
Grippe-like	Fever, chills, malaise, headache, myalgia, eye pain, hyperaesthesias	Brucellosis Chickungunya fever Dengue fever Influenza Inhalation anthrax (early) Q-fever Rift Valley fever Venezuelan equine encephalitis

Syndrome	General Characteristics	Potential Causes
Hemorrhagic Fever	Fever; hypotension, with or without fever	Argentine hemorrhagic fever Bolivian hemorrhagic fever Crimean-Congo hemorrhagic fever Dengue fever Ebola/Marburg Korean hemorrhagic fever Lassa fever Omsk hemorrhagic fever Plague Rift Valley fever (infrequent) Smallpox Trichothecene mycotoxins Yellow fever
Jaundice	With or without fever	Ebola/Marburg Lassa fever Toxins (especially aflatoxin) Yellow fever

Syndrome	General Characteristics	Potential Causes
Oliguric renal failure	Typically with fever	Korean hemorrhagic fever Psittacosis (rarely) Yellow fever
Pharyngitis	Sore throat, dysphagia, with or without fever	Botulinum toxins Ebola/Marburg Lassa fever Ricin Trichothecene mycotoxins Tularemia
Polyarthritis/ polyarthralgia	Typically with fever	Chickungunya fever

Syndrome	General Characteristics	Potential Causes
Pulmonary syndrome	Pneumonia, respiratory insufficiency, respiratory distres, usually with fever	Anthrax Botulinum toxin Coccidiodornycosis Crimean-Congo hemorrhagic fever Clostridium perfringens toxins Histoplasmosis Influenza Korean hemorrhagic fever Omsk hemorrhagic fever Plague Psittacosis Q-fever Ricin Staphylococcus enterotoxin B Tularemia

Syndrome	General Characteristics	Potential Causes
Rapid death syndrome	Death within minutes; fever may be present	Botulinum toxins Chemical agents Saxitoxin Tetradotoxin Trichothecene mycotoxins Other toxins
Rash-maculopapular	All rash syndromes typically accompanied by fever	Argentine hemorrhagic fever Bolivian hemorrhagic fever Chickungunya fever Dengue fever Ebola/Marburg Epidemic typhus Psittacosis (uncommon) Rocky Mountain spotted fever Scrub typhus Smallpox (early) Tularemia (uncommon)

Syndrome	General Characteristics	Potential Causes
Rash-petechial/ecchymotic		Argentine hemorrhagic fever Bolivian hemorrhagic fever Crimean-Congo hemorrhagic fever Dengue fever Ebola/Marburg Epidemic typhus Korean hemorrhagic fever Lassa fever Omsk hemorrhagic fever Plague Rift Valley fever (infrequent) Scrub typhus Smallpox (rare, fulminant) Trichothecene mycotoxins Yellow fever

Syndrome	General Characteristics	Potential Causes
Rash-vesiculopustular		Meliaidosis Smallpox Tularemia
Rash-granulomatous or uberative		Meliaidosis Tularemia
Stiff neck syndrome	Typically with fever	Eastern equine encephalitis Histoplasmosis Psittacosis Venezuelan equine encephalitis Western equine encephalitis

B-2 - Bacteria

Bacteria are unicellular organisms. They vary in shape and size from spherical cells - cocci - with a diameter of 0.5-1.0 (m (micrometer), to long rod-shaped organisms - bacilli - which may be from 1-5 (m in size. Chains of bacilli may exceed 50 (m. The shape of the bacterial cell is determined by the rigid cell wall. The interior of the cell contains the nuclear material (DNA), cytoplasm, and cell membrane, which are necessary for the life of the bacterium. Many bacteria also have glycoproteins on their outer surfaces which aid in bacterial attachment to surface receptors on cells and are of special importance in their ability to cause disease. Under special circumstances some types of bacteria can transform into spores. The spore of the bacterial cell is more resistant to cold, heat, drying, chemicals and radiation than the bacterium itself. Spores are a dormant form of the bacterium and, like the seeds of plants, they can germinate when conditions are favorable.

Bacteria can cause diseases in human beings and animals by means of two mechanisms that differ in principle: in one case by invading the tissues, in the other by producing poisons (toxins). In many cases pathogenic bacteria possess both properties. The diseases they produce often respond to specific therapy with antibiotics.

Notes:

Anthrax
(Bacillus anthracis)

Signs and Symptoms:
- Three forms in man:
    - Cutaneous – black carbuncles or swelling at the site of infection.
    - Inhalational
    - Gastrointestinal
- Incubation period 1-6 days.
- Fever, malaise, fatigue, cough and mild chest discomfort is followed by severe respiratory distress with dyspnea, diaphoresis, stridor, and cyanosis.
- Initial symptoms often followed by a short period of improvement (hours to 2-3 days).
- Shock and death occurs within 24-36 hours of severe symptoms.

Diagnosis:
- Physical findings are non-specific.
- Possible widened mediastinum.
- Detectable by Gram stain of blood and by blood culture late in course of illness.

Treatment:
- Usually not effective after symptoms are manifested.
- Penicillin, tetracyclines (doxycycline), erythromycin, chloramphenicol, gentamicin or ciprofloxacin
- Supportive therapy

Decontamination and Precautions:
- Sporicidal agent (iodine or chlorine).

Notes:

Brucellosis
(Brucella melitensis)

Signs and Symptoms:
- Incubation period is quite variable, normally ranging from 3-4 weeks, but may be as short as 1 week or as long as several months.
- Acute and subacute brucellosis are quite non-specific and consist of irregular fever, headache, profound weakness and fatigue, chills and sweating, and generalized arthralgias and myalgias
- Cough occurs in 15-25%, but the chest x-ray usually is normal.
- Untreated disease can persist for months to years, often with relapses and remissions.
- Fatalities are uncommon, even in the absence of therapy.

Diagnosis:
- Initial symptoms of brucellosis are usually nonspecific, differential diagnosis is very broad and includes bacterial,

viral, and mycoplasmal infections

• Systemic symptoms of brucellosis may persist for prolonged periods.

• Brucellosis may be indistinguishable clinically from the typhoidal form of tularemia or from typhoid fever itself.

• Brucellae may be isolated from standard blood cultures, but require a prolonged period of incubation; cultures should thus be maintained for six weeks if brucellosis is suspected.

Treatment:

• Recommended treatment is doxycycline (200 mg/day) plus rifampin (900 mg/day) for 6 weeks.

• Alternative effective treatment consists of doxycycline (200 mg/day) for 6 weeks plus streptomycin (1 gm/day) for 3 weeks.

Decontamination and Precautions:

• Surfaces contaminated with brucella aerosols may be decontaminated by standard means (0.5% hypochlorite).

• Drainage and secretion precautions should be practiced in patients who have open skin lesions; otherwise no evidence of person-to-person transmission of brucellosis exists.

Notes:

• Under selected environmental conditions (for example, darkness, cool temperatures, high CO_2), persistence for up to 2 years has been documented
• Most likely be delivered by the aerosol route
• Infection caused by one of four species of Gram-negative coccobacilli of the genus Brucella.
• B. abortus (cattle), B. melitensis, (goats & camels), B. suis (pigs), and B. canis (dogs)

Cholera
(Vibrio cholerae)

Signs and Symptoms:
- Incubation period is 12-72 hours.
- Asymptomatic to severe with sudden onset.
- Vomiting, headache, intestinal cramping with little or no fever followed rapidly by painless, voluminous diarrhea. Fluid losses may exceed 5 to 10 liters per day.
- Without treatment, death may result from severe dehydration, hypovolemia and shock.

Diagnosis:
- Clinical diagnosis - 'Rice water' diarrhea and dehydration.
- Microscopic exam of stool samples reveals few or no red or white cells. Can be identified by darkfield or phase contrast microscopy, and by direct visualization of darting motile vibrio.

Treatment:
- Fluid and electrolyte replacement.
- Antibiotics (tetracycline, ciprofloxacin or erythromycin) will shorten the duration of diarrhea and shedding of the organism.

Decontamination and Precautions:
- Personal contact rarely causes infection; however, enteric precautions and careful hand-washing should be employed.
- Bacteriocidal solutions (hypochlorite) would provide adequate decontamination.

Notes:

Plague
(Yersinia pestis)

Signs and Symptoms:

Pneumonic plague:
- Incubation period is 2-3 days.
- High fever, chills, headache, hemoptysis, and toxemia, progressing rapidly to dyspnea, stridor, and cyanosis. Death results from respiratory failure, circulatory collapse, and a bleeding diathesis.

Bubonic plague:
- Incubation period is 2-10 days.
- Malaise, high fever, and tender lymph nodes (buboes); may progress spontaneously to the septicemic form, with spread to the CNS, lungs, and elsewhere.

Diagnosis:
- Clinical diagnosis - A presumptive diagnosis can be made by Gram or Wayson stain of lymph node aspirates,

sputum, or CSF.
• Plague can also be cultured.

Treatment and Isolation:
   • Early administration of antibiotics is very effective. Supportive therapy for pneumonic and septicemic forms is required.
   • Strict isolation of patients with pneumonic plague.

Decontamination and Precautions:
   • Secretion and lesion precautions with bubonic plague.
   • Heat, disinfectants and exposure to sunlight renders bacteria harmless.

Notes:

Tularemia
(Francisella tularensis)

Signs and Symptoms:
- Ulceroglandular tularemia presents with a local ulcer and regional lymphaden opathy, fever, chills, headache and malaise.
- Typhoidal or septicemic tularemia presents with fever, headache, malaise, substernal discomfort, prostration, weight loss and a non-productive cough.

Diagnosis:
- Clinical diagnosis - Physical findings are usually non-specific. Chest x-ray may reveal a pneumonic process, mediastinal lymphadenopathy or pleural effusion.
- Routine culture is possible but difficult.
- The diagnosis can be established retrospectively by serology.

Treatment and Isolation:
- Administration of antibiotics (streptomycin or gentamicin) with early treatment is very effective.
- Strict isolation of patients is not required.

Decontamination and Precautions:
- Secretion and lesion precautions should be practiced.
- Organisms are relatively easy to render harmless by heat and disinfectants.

Notes:

Q Fever
(Coxiella burnetii)

Signs and Symptoms:
- Fever, cough, and pleuritic chest pain may occur as early as ten days after exposure.
- Patients are not generally critically ill, and the illness lasts from 2 days to 2 weeks.

Diagnosis:
- Q Fever is not a clinically distinct illness and may resemble a viral illness or other types of atypical pneumonia.
- The diagnosis is confirmed serologically.

Treatment:
- Q Fever is generally a self-limited illness even without treatment.
- Tetracycline or doxycycline are the treatments of choice and are given orally for 5 to 7 days.
- Q Fever endocarditis (rare) is much

more difficult to treat.

Decontamination and Precautions:
• Patients who are exposed to Q Fever by aerosol do not present a risk for secondary contamination or re-aerosolization of the organism.
• Decontamination is accomplished with soap and water or by the use of weak (0.5%) hypochlorite solutions.

Notes:

Toxins are chemical by-products produced by plants, animals, or microorganisms. It is the chemicals that cause injury not the organisms that make the toxins.

Important Notes:
- Toxins do not grow, reproduce, or die after they have been dispersed.
- Field monitors capable of rapid detection are not available.
- Toxins produce effects similar to those caused by chemical agents.
- Toxins can penetrate the unbroken skin.
- Symptoms of an attack may appear very rapidly.
- Very small doses will cause injuries and/or death.
- Time from exposure to onset of clinical signs may also vary greatly among toxins.

Therapy:

- Specific antitoxins are available for certain conditions.
- No broad-spectrum antitoxins currently exist.

Notes:

Botulinum toxin

Signs and Symptoms:
• Ptosis, generalized weakness, dizziness, dry mouth and throat, blurred vision and diplopia, dysarthria, dysphonia, and dysphagia followed by symmetrical descending flaccid paralysis and development of respiratory failure.
• Symptoms begin as early as 24-36 hours but may take several days after inhalation of toxin.

Diagnosis:
• Clinical diagnosis - No routine laboratory findings.
• Biowarfare attack should be suspected if numerous collocated casualties have progressive descending bulbar, muscular, and respiratory weakness.

Treatment:
• Intubation and ventilatory assistance for respiratory failure.
• Tracheostomy may be required.

Administration of botulinum antitoxin (IND product) may prevent or decrease progression to respiratory failure and hasten recovery.

Decontamination and Precautions:
• Hypochlorite (0.5% for 10-15 minutes) and/or soap and water.
• Toxin is not dermally active and secondary aerosols are not a hazard from patients.

Source:
• Bacteria (Clostridium botulinum)

Notes:

Ricin

Signs and Symptoms:

• Weakness, fever, cough and pulmonary edema occur 18-24 hours after inhalation exposure, followed by severe respiratory distress and death from hypoxemia in 36-72 hours.

Diagnosis:

• Signs and symptoms noted above in large numbers of geographically clustered patients could suggest an exposure to aerosolized ricin.

• The rapid time course to severe symptoms and death would be unusual for infectious agents.

• Laboratory findings are nonspecific but similar to other pulmonary irritants which cause pulmonary edema. Specific serum ELISA is available. Acute and convalescent sera should be collected.

Treatment:
- Management is supportive and should include treatment for pulmonary edema.
- Gastric decontamination measures should be used if ingested.

Decontamination and Precautions:
- Weak hypochlorite solutions and/or soap and water can decontaminate skin surfaces.
- Ricin is not volatile, so secondary aerosols are generally not a danger to health care providers.

Source:
- Seed ("bean") of the castor plant.
- Over 1 million tons of castor "beans" are processed annually worldwide in the production of castor oil.

Notes:

Saxitoxin

Signs and Symptoms:
• Symptoms typically begin 10-60 minutes after exposure.

• Symptoms may be delayed several hours depending upon the dose and individual idiosyncrasy.

• Initial symptoms include numbness or tingling of the lips, tongue and fingertips, followed by numbness of the neck and extremities and general muscular incoordination.

• Nausea and vomiting may be present, other symptoms may include a feeling of light headedness, or floating, dizziness, weakness, aphasia, incoherence, visual disturbances, memory loss and headache.

• Respiratory distress and flaccid muscular paralysis are the terminal stages and can occur 2-12 hours after intoxication.

• Death results from respiratory paralysis.

• Clearance of the toxin is rapid and survivors for 12-24 hours will usually recover.
• Complete recovery may require 7-14 days.

Diagnosis:

• Differential diagnosis may require toxin detection.
• Diagnosis is confirmed by detection of toxin in the food, water, stomach contents or environmental samples.
• Saxitoxin, neosaxitoxin, and several other derivatives can be detected by ELISA or by mouse bioassay.

Treatment:

• Management is supportive and standard management of poison ingestion should be employed if intoxication is by the oral route.
• Toxins are rapidly cleared and excreted in the urine, so diuresis may increase

elimination.
• Intubation and mechanical respiratory support may be required in severe intoxication.
• Specific antitoxin therapy has been successful in animal models, but is untested in humans.

Decontamination and Precautions:
• Hypochlorite (0.5% for 10-15 minutes) and/or soap and water.
• Secondary aerosols are not a hazard from patients.

Notes:
• Rapidly absorbed

Staphylococcal enterotoxin B

Signs and Symptoms:
- From 3-12 hours after exposure.
- Sudden onset of fever, chills, headache, diarrhea, nausea, vomiting, muscle aches, shortness of breath, and nonproductive cough.
- Some patients may develop shortness of breath and retrosternal chest pain.
- Fever may last 2-5 days, and cough may persist for up to 4 weeks.
- Patients may also present with nausea, vomiting, and diarrhea if they swallow toxin.
- Higher exposure can lead to septic shock and death.

Diagnosis:
- Diagnosis is clinical.
- Patients present with a febrile respiratory syndrome without CXR abnormalities.
- Large numbers of victims presenting with typical symptoms and signs of SEB

pulmonary exposure would suggest an intentional attack with this toxin.

Treatment:
- Treatment is limited to supportive care.
- Artificial ventilation might be needed for very severe cases, and attention to fluid management is important.

Decontamination and Precautions:
- Hypochlorite (0.5% for 10-15 minutes) and/or soap and water.
- Destroy any food that may have been contaminated.

Notes:
- Causes illness at extremely low doses, but relatively high doses are required to kill.

Source:
- Bacteria (Staphylococcus)

Trichothecene mycotoxins (T2)

Signs and Symptoms:
  • Exposure causes skin pain, pruritus, redness, vesicles, necrosis and sloughing of epidermis.
  • Effects on the airway include nose and throat pain, nasal discharge, itching and sneezing, cough, dyspnea, wheezing, chest pain and hemoptysis.
  • Also produces effects after ingestion or eye contact.
  • Severe poisoning results in prostration, weakness, ataxia, collapse, shock, and death.

Diagnosis:
  • "Yellow rain" with droplets of yellow fluid contaminating clothes and the environment.
  • Confirmation requires testing of blood, tissue and environmental samples.

Treatment:
  • No specific antidote.

• Superactivated charcoal should be given orally if swallowed.

Decontamination:
- Soap and water
- Eye exposure treated with copious saline irrigation
- Sodium hydroxide and sodium hypochlorite will detoxify.

Source:
- Fungi

Notes:
- One of the more stable toxins, retaining its bioactivity even when heated to high temperatures.
- Unlike most toxins, T-2 is dermally active.

Viruses are the simplest type of microorganism and consist of a nucleocapsid protein coat containing genetic material, either RNA or DNA. In some cases an outer layer of lipids also surrounds the virus particle. Viruses are much smaller than bacteria and vary in size from 0.02 (m to 0.2 (m (1 (m = 1/1000 mm). Viruses lack a system for their own metabolism and are therefore dependent on their host cells: viruses are thus intracellular parasites. This also means that the virus, unlike the bacterium, cannot be cultivated in synthetic nutritive solutions but requires living cells in order to multiply. The host cells can be from human beings, animals, plants, or bacteria. Every virus needs its own special type of host cell because a complicated interaction is required between the cell and virus if the virus is to be able to multiply. Many virus-specific host cells can be cultivated in synthetic nutrient solutions and afterwards can be infected with the virus in question. The cultivation of viruses is a costly, demanding, and time-consuming process. A virus normally brings about changes in the host cell such that the cell dies.

Antiviral Therapy:

- The only "broad-spectrum" antiviral drug currently available is ribavirin.
- Other antiviral drugs, such as amantadine, acyclovir, and azidothymidine, are restricted in their therapeutic spectrum to single virus families, and thus have little application as non-specific antivirals.

Venezuelan Equine Encephalitis

Signs and Symptoms:
- Sudden onset of illness with generalized malaise, spiking fevers, rigors, severe headache, photophobia, and myalgias.
- Nausea, vomiting, cough, sore throat, and diarrhea may follow.
- Full recovery takes 1-2 weeks.

Diagnosis:
- Clinical diagnosis. Physical findings are usually non-specific.
- The white blood cell count often shows a striking leukopenia and lymphopenia.
- Virus isolation may be made from serum, and in some cases throat swab specimens.

Treatment:
- Supportive only.

Decontamination and Precautions:

- Blood and body fluid precautions should be practiced.
- Human cases are infectious for mosquitoes for at least 72 hours.
- The virus can be destroyed by heat (80 degrees centigrade for 30 minutes) and ordinary disinfectants.

Notes:

Viral Hemorrhagic Fevers

Viral Hemorrhagic fevers (VHF) comprise a group of viruses categorized by the clinical syndrom they may cause in humans. FILOVIRIDAE, which consists of Ebola and Marburg viruses; the ARENAVIRIDAE, including Lassa fever, Argentine and Bolivian hemorrhagic fever viruses; the BUNYAVIRIDAE, including various members from the Hantavirus genus, Congo-Crimean hemorrhagic fever virus from the Nairovirus genus, and Rift Valley fever from the Phlebovirus genus; and FLAVIVIRIDAE, such as Yellow fever virus and Dengue hemorrhagic fever virus]

Signs and Symptoms:

- VHFs are febrile illnesses which can be complicated by easy bleeding, petechiae, hypotension and even shock, flushing of the face and chest, and edema.
- Constitutional symptoms such as malaise, myalgias, headache, vomiting,

and diarrhea may occur in any of the hemorrhagic fevers.

• Full-blown VHF typically evolves to shock and generalized mucous membrane hemorrhage and often is accompanied by evidence of neurologic, hematopoietic, or pulmonary involvement.

Diagnosis:

• Definitive diagnosis rests on specific virologic techniques.

• Most patients have readily detectable viremia at presentation (exception: hantaviral infections).

• Not all infected patients develop VHF

• Rapid enzyme immunoassays can detect viral antigens in acute sera from patients with Lassa, Argentine HF, Rift Valley fever, Congo-Crimean HF, yellow fever and specific IgM antibodies in early convalescence.

• Diagnosis by virus cultivation and identification will require 3-10 days or longer.

• Significant numbers of patients with a hemorrhagic fever syndrome should suggest the diagnosis of a viral hemorrhagic fever.
• For much of the world, the major differential diagnosis is malaria.

Treatment and Isolation:

• Intensive supportive care may be required.
• Antiviral therapy with ribavirin may be useful in several of these infections.
• Convalescent plasma may be effective in Argentine hemorrhagic fever.
• Isolation measures and barrier procedures are indicated.

Decontamination and Precautions:

• Decontamination with hypochlorite or phenolic disinfectants.

Notes:

• Evidence for weaponization does not exist for many of these viruses.
• The viruses may be spread in a variety

of ways, and for some there is a possibility that humans could be infected through a respiratory portal of entry.

• All of these viruses (except for dengue virus) are infectious by aerosol or fomites.

• Potential for nosocomial transmission to patients, medical staff, and other response personnel (except Hantavirus infections).

• Special caution must be exercised in handling sharps, needles, and other potential sources of parenteral exposure.

• Caution should be exercised in evaluating and treating the patient with a suspected VHF.

SECTION C

Chemical Agents

C-1 - Introduction

C-2 - Nerve Agents

C-3 - Blister Agents

C-4 - Choking Agents

C-5 - Blood Agents

C-6 - Vomiting Agents

C-1 - Introduction

Chemical Agents:
This section will help identify chemical agents.

There are five categories of chemical agents:
- Nerve
- Blister
- Choking
- Blood
- Vomiting

Each chemical agent is divided into six essential elements as follows:
Characteristics:
- Descriptive elements:
    - Color
    - Odor
    - Consistency
- Physical state:
    - Vapor
    - Aerosol
    - Liquid.

- Ability to remain in environment – persistent or non-persistent.

Toxicology:
- Median incapacitating dosage
- Median lethal dosage

Physical Findings:
- Clinical symptomology

Protection Required:
- Personal Protective Equipment (PPE)
- Immediate action if exposed to an agent

Medical Management:
- Antidotes
- Treatments

Decontamination:
- Type of decontamination
  - Chemical destruction
  - Physical removal
  - Sealing
  - Neutralization

Notes:

VX

Characteristics:
- Amber-colored, oily, odorless liquid
- Inhibits acetylcholinesterase, disrupting nerve impulse transmission.
- Persistent – remains on ground for weeks (longer in cold weather).
- Primarily a liquid hazard.
- Dispersed in liquid, aerosol, or vapor form.

Toxicology:
- Median Incapacitating dosage – 50 mg-min/m^3
- Median Lethal dosage – 100 mg-min/m^3
- Clinical symptoms gradual or rapid depending exposure.
- Easily absorbed through skin or eyes.

Physical Findings:

Liquid Small to Moderate Exposure	**Liquid** Large Exposure	**Vapor** Small to Moderate Exposure	**Vapor** Large Exposure
Localized Sweating	Sweating	Miosis	Sweating
Nausea	Lacrimation	Rhinorrhea	Lacrimation
Vomiting	Urination	Mild Difficulty Breathing	Urination
Feeling of Weakness	Diarrhea		Diarrhea
	Gasping		Gasping
	Epilepsy (seizures)		Epilepsy (seizures)
			Miosis

C-2-89

VX

Protection Required:

- Long-term contact hazard from contaminated ground, vegetation and equipment possible.
- Protective mask and protective clothing
- Decontamination of clothing and skin if VX exposure suspected.

Medical Management:

- Atropine – 2mg i.v. at 5-10 min intervals for total of 8mg
- Pralidoxime chloride – 600mg i.v. at 5-10 min intervals for total of 1600mg
- Diazepam – 10mg i.v. at 10 min intervals or Ativan – 2-4 mg for convulsing casualty.
- Ventilation and supportive therapy

Decontamination:

- Aqueous hypochlorite solution (household bleach)
- Large amounts of water.

Sarin (GB)

Characteristics:
- Colorless, odorless liquid.
- Mixes readily with water.
- Inhibits acetylcholinesterase, disrupting nerve impulse transmission.
- Non-persistent – evaporates rapidly
- Primarily dispersed in an aerosol or vapor form.

Toxicology:
- Median Incapacitating dosage (unmasked) – 75 mg-min/m^3 (resting personnel)
- Median Lethal dosage – 100 mg-min/m^3 (resting personnel)
- Clinical symptoms gradual or rapid depending on amount of exposure.
- Rapidly absorbed through respiratory tract.
- Onset of toxicity within several minutes to a few hours depending on concentration of agent.

GB

Physical Findings:

Low Concentration	High Concentration
Miosis	Cough
Headache	Difficulty Breathing
Increased Salivation	Increased Sweating
Rhinorrhea	Nausea
Bronchoconstriction	Vomiting
	Cramps
	Diarrhea
	Muscular Twitching
	Death by suffocation

Protection Required:

• If Sarin is not immediately vaporized it can form a contact hazard which can subsequently reinforce the respiratory hazard.

• Increased lethality at higher environmental temperatures (especially through skin).

• Protective mask and protective clothing.

GB   C-2-92

• Immediate decontamination of clothes and skin if Sarin exposure suspected. (Clothes give off GB agent for 30 minutes after contact).

Medical Management:
• Atropine – 2mg i.v. at 5-10 min intervals for total of 8mg
• Pralidoxime chloride – 600mg i.v. at 5-10 min intervals for total of 1600mg
• Diazepam – 10mg i.v. at 10 min intervals or Ativan – 2-4 mg i.v. for convulsing casualty.
• Ventilation and supportive therapy

Decontamination:
• Alkaline solutions accelerate decomposition.
• Aqueous hypochlorite solution (household bleach)
• Large amounts of water.
• An area exposed to Sarin will decontaminate itself within a few days.

Tabun (GA)

Characteristics:
- Colorless to brownish liquid giving a colorless vapor.
- Reacts slowly with water but rapidly with strong acids and alkalies.
- Faintly fruity odor unless pure.
- Inhibits acetylcholinesterase, disrupting nerve impulse transmission.
- Persistence, 1-2 days under average weather conditions.
- Primarily dispersed in an aerosol or vapor form.

Toxicology:
- Median Incapacitating dosage (unmasked) – 300 mg-min/m^3 (resting personnel)
- Median Lethal dosage – 400 mg-min/m^3 (resting personnel)
- Respiratory lethal dosages kill in 1-10 min.

- Large amount on skin may cause death in 1-2 min.
- Number and severity of symptoms dependant on quantity and rate of entry into body.

Physical Findings:

Low Concentration	High Concentration
Miosis	Cough
Headache	Difficulty Breathing
Increased Salivation	Increased Sweating
Rhinorrhea	Nausea
Bronchoconstriction	Vomiting
	Cramps
	Diarrhea
	Muscular Twitching
	Death by suffocation

Protection Required:
- Protective mask and protective clothing
- Immediate decon of clothes (Clothes give off GA agent for 30 min.)

GA

Medical Management:
- Atropine – 2mg i.v. at 5-10 min intervals for total of 8mg
- Pralidoxime chloride – 600mg i.v. at 5-10 min intervals for total of 1600mg
- Diazepam – 10mg i.v. at 10 min intervals or Ativan – 2-4 mg i.v. for convulsing casualty.
- Ventilation and supportive therapy

Decontamination:
- Bleach slurry
- Dilute alkali solutions
- Steam and ammonia in a confined area.
- Hot soapy water

Notes:

Soman (GD)

Characteristics:
- Industrial product-yellow-brown liquid camphor-like odor.
- Colorless liquid when pure-fruity odor.
- Mixes readily with water.
- Inhibits acetylcholinesterase, disrupting nerve impulse transmission.
- Non-persistent – evaporates rapidly
- Primarily dispersed in an aerosol or vapor form.

Toxicology:
- Median Incapacitating dosage (unmasked) – 75 to 300 mg-min/m³ (resting personnel)
- Median Lethal dosage – 100 to 400 mg-min/m³ (resting personnel)
- Rapidly absorbed through respiratory tract.
- Onset of toxicity within several minutes to a few hours depending on concentration of agent.

Physical Findings:

Low Concentration	High Concentration
Miosis	Cough
Headache	Difficulty Breathing
Increased Salivation	Increased Sweating
Rhinorrhea	Nausea
Bronchoconstriction	Vomiting
	Cramps
	Diarrhea
	Muscular Twitching
	Death by suffocation

Protection Required:

- Increased lethality at higher environmental temperatures (especially through skin).
- Protective mask and protective clothing.
- Immediate decontamination of clothes and skin if Soman exposure suspected.

GD   C-2-98

(Clothes give off GD agent for 30 minutes after contact).

Medical Management:
- Atropine – 2mg i.v. at 5-10 min intervals for total of 8mg
- Pralidoxime chloride – 600mg i.v. at 5-10 min intervals for total of 1600mg
- Diazepam – 10mg i.v. at 10 min intervals or Ativan – 2-4 mg i.v. for convulsing casualty.
- Ventilation and supportive therapy

Decontamination:
- Solids, powders and solutions containing various types of bleach.
- Towelettes moistened with NaOH dissolved in water, phenol, ethanol, and ammonia.

Notes:

GD

Distilled Mustard (HD)

Characteristics:
- Oily liquid with color ranging from light yellow to brown.
- Water clear if pure.
- Odor of garlic, onion or mustard.
- Primarily a liquid hazard.
- Vapor hazard increases with increasing temperature (100 degrees Fahrenheit or above).
- First symptoms appear in 4-6 hrs.

Toxicology:
- Median Incapacitating dosage:
  - Eye injury – 200 mg-min/m^3
  - Skin absorption – 2,000 mg-min/m^3
- Median Lethal dosage:
  - Inhalation – 1,500 mg-min/m^3
  - Skin absorption – 10,000 mg-min/m^3
- Wet skin absorbs more mustard than dry.
- Exerts casualty effect at lower

HD

concentration in hot humid weather.
• Repeated exposures are cumulative.

Physical Findings:

Organ/System	Symptomology
Skin	Erythema appears in 2-24 hrs. Large, dome-shaped, thin-walled, translucent, yellowish blisters. Blister fluid clear but does not contain mustard.
Eyes	Low dose vapor exposure irritation: • Reddening of the eyes High dose vapor exposure: • Severe conjunctivitis • Photophobia • Blepharospasm • Pain • Corneal damage
Pulmonary	Hoarseness Loss of voice Productive cough Fever Dysnea Moist rhonchi and rales

HD

Gastrointestinal (food & water contaminated by liquid mustard)	Nausea Vomiting Pain Diarrhea Prostration
Central Nervous System	Apathy Depression Intellectual Dullness
Metabolism	Death in 5-10 days. Pulmonary insufficiency Compromised immune response.

Protection Required:
- Protective mask
- Permeable protective clothing for vapor and small droplets.
- Impermeable clothing for large droplets, splashes and smears.
- Immediate decontamination of clothes and skin if Mustard exposure suspected.

Medical Management:
- Skin
- Immediate decon of affected area.

- Unroof blisters and clean
- Topical antibiotics
- Silver sulfadiazine
- Sulfamylon
- Bacitracin
- Neosporin
- Eyes
- Immediate irrigation with large amounts of water.
- Supportive therapy

Decontamination:
- Sodium hypochlorite solution.
- Large amounts of water.

Notes:

Nitrogen Mustard (HN)

Characteristics:
- Oily, colorless to pale yellow liquid.
- Partially soluble in water.
- Freely soluble in organic solvents.
- Faint fishy or musty odor.
- Liquid or vapor form
- First symptoms in 12 hrs or longer.

Toxicology:
- Median Incapacitating dosage:
  - Eye injury – 200 mg-min/m^3
  - Skin absorption (masked) – 9,000 mg-min/m^3
- Median Lethal dosage:
  - Inhalation – 1,500 mg-min/m^3
  - Skin absorption (masked) – 20,000 mg-min/m^3

Physical Findings:

Organ/System	Symptomology
Skin	Erythema appears in 2-24 hrs. Large, dome-shaped, thin-walled, translucent, yellowish blisters. Blister fluid clear but does not contain mustard.
Eyes	Low dose vapor exposure irritation: • Reddening of the eyes High dose vapor exposure: • Severe conjunctivitis • Photophobia • Blepharospasm • Pain • Corneal damage
Pulmonary	Hoarseness Loss of voice Productive cough Fever Dysnea Moist rhonchi and rales
Gastrointestinal (food & water contaminated by liquid mustard)	Nausea Vomiting Pain Diarrhea Prostration

HN

Protection Required:

- Protective mask
- Permeable protective clothing for vapor and small droplets.
- Impermeable clothing for large droplets, splashes and smears.
- Immediate decontamination of clothes and skin if Nitrogen Mustard exposure suspected.

Medical Management:

- Skin
- Immediate decontamination of affected area.
- Unroof blisters and clean
- Topical antibiotics
- Silver sulfadiazine
- Sulfamylon
- Bacitracin
- Neosporin
- Eyes
- Immediate irrigation with large amounts of water.
- Supportive therapy

Decontamination:
- Supertropical bleach (STB)
- Large amounts of water.
- Fire

Notes:

Sulfur Mustard (H)

Characteristics:
- Oily liquid with a color ranging from light yellow to brown.
- Odor of garlic, onion, or mustard.
- Evaporates slowly
- Primarily a liquid hazard.
- Vapor hazard increases with temperature (100 degrees F or above).
- Mustard reacts with tissue in minutes of entering body.
- Blood, tissue, blister fluid do not contain mustard.

Toxicology:
- Median Incapacitating dosage:
  - Eye injury – 200 mg-min/m^3
  - Skin absorption – 2000 mg-min/m^3
- Median Lethal dosage:
  - Inhalation – 1500 mg-min/m^3
  - Skin absorption – 10,000 mg-min/m^3
- Wet skin absorbs more mustard than dry.
- Exerts casualty effect at lower

concentration in hot humid weather.
• Repeated exposures are cumulative.

Physical Findings:

Organ/System	Symptomology
Skin	Erythema appears in 2-24 hrs. Large, dome-shaped, thin-walled, translucent, yellowish blisters. Blister fluid clear but does not contain mustard.
Eyes	Low dose vapor exposure irritation: • Reddening of the eyes High dose vapor exposure: • Severe conjunctivitis • Photophobia • Blepharospasm • Pain • Corneal damage
Pulmonary	Hoarseness Loss of voice Productive cough Fever Dysnea Moist rhonchi and rales

H

Gastrointestinal (food & water contaminated by liquid mustard)	Nausea Vomiting Pain Diarrhea Prostration
Central Nervous System	Apathy Depression Intellectual Dullness
Metabolism	Death in 5-10 days. Pulmonary insufficiency Compromised immune response.

Protection Required:
- Protective mask
- Permeable protective clothing for vapor and small droplets.
- Impermeable clothing for large droplets, splashes and smears.
- Immediate decontamination of clothes and skin if Mustard exposure suspected.

Medical Management:
- Skin
- Immediate decon of affected area.

- Unroof blisters and clean
- Topical antibiotics
- Silver sulfadiazine
- Sulfamylon
- Bacitracin
- Neosporin
- Eyes
- Immediate irrigation with large amounts of water.
- Supportive therapy

Decontamination:
- Sodium hypochlorite solution
- Large amounts of water.

Notes:

H

Phosgene Oxime (CX)

Characteristics:
- Disagreeable, penetrating odor.
- Appears as liquid or colorless solid.
- Readily soluble in water.
- Liquid or vapor causes pain on contact.
- Corrodes most metals.

Toxicology:
- Median Incapacitating dosage:
    - Eye injury (from vapor) – below 300 mg-min/m³
    - Skin absorption (masked personnel) – over 1,500 mg-min/m³
- Median Lethal dosage:
    - Inhalation (unmasked) – 1500-2000 mg-min/m³
    - Skin absorption (masked personnel) – 100,000 mg-min/m³

Physical Findings:

Organ/System	Symptomology
Skin	Blanching with erthematous ring in 30 seconds. Wheal in 30 minutes. Necrosis later.
Eyes	Extreme pain Permanent loss of sight if not decontaminated.
Pulmonary	Irritating to upper airway. Pulmonary edema after inhalation and skin application.
Gastrointestinal	Hemorrahagic inflammatory changes.

Protection Required:

- Protective mask
- Protective clothing for body.
- Immediate decontamination of clothes and skin if Phosgene Oxime exposure suspected.

Medical Management:
- Immediate decontamination
- Symptomatic management of lesions.

Decontamination:
- Large amounts of water.

Notes:

Lewisite (L)

Characteristics:
- Effects similar to HD.
- Acts as systematic poison.
- Immediate pain
- Geranium-like odor
- Little odor when pure.
- Rapid rate of action.

Toxicology:
- Median Incapacitating dosage:
  - Eye injury (from vapor) – <300 mg-min/m^3
  - Skin absorption (masked personnel) – >1500 mg-min/m^3
- Median Lethal dosage:
  - Inhalation (unmasked) – 1200 to 1500 mg-min/m^3
  - Skin absorption (masked personnel) – 100,000 mg-min/m^3

L

Physical Findings:

Systematic Poison	Liquid
Pulmonary edema	Immediate eye pain
Diarrhea	Loss of sight unless decontaminated within 1 minute.
Restlessness	Immediate skin pain
Weakness	Reddening of skin within 30 minutes.
Subnormal temperature	Blistering in 13 hours.
Low blood pressure	

Protection Required:
- Protective mask
- Permeable protective clothing for vapor and small droplets.

L

- Impermeable clothing for large droplets, splashes and smears.
- Immediate decontamination of clothes and skin if Lewisite exposure suspected.

Medical Management:
- Immediate decontamination
- Symptomatic management of lesions.
- Specific Antidote – British Anti-Lewisite (BAL)
- Intramuscular for systematic effects.
- BAL skin ointment – decrease severity of skin lesions
- BAL ophthalmic Ointment - decrease severity of eye lesions

Decontamination:
- Hypochlorite solution
- Caustic soda
- Large amounts of water.

Notes:

L

Phenyldichloroarsine (PD)

Characteristics:
- Colorless to brown liquids.
- Soluble in most organic solvents but poorly in water.
- More volatile than mustard.
- No odor
- As liquid penetrates rubber and most impermeable fabrics.
- Immediate effect on eyes.
- Skin delayed 30 minutes to 1 hour.
- Persistency – shorter than HD

Toxicology:
- Median detectable concentration – nasal and throat irritation.
- Median Incapacitating dosage:
    - Vomiting agent – 16 mg-min/m^3
    - Blistering agent – 1,800 mg-min/m^3
- Median Lethal dosage:
    - Inhalation – 2,600 mg-min/m^3

Physical Findings:

Organ/System	Symptomology
Skin	Erythema Thick roofed blisters Yellowish blister fluid - nontoxic
Eyes	Pain and blepharospasm occur instantly. Edema of conjunctivae and lids.
Pulmonary	Pulmonary edema
Systemic	Systemic poisoning Acute poisoning result in hypovolemic shock.

Protection Required:

- Protective mask
- Permeable protective clothing for vapor and small droplets.
- Impermeable clothing for large

PD

droplets, splashes and smears.

Medical Management:
- BAL ointment – skin
- Morphine – pain
- Atropine sulfate ointment – eyes
- Intramuscular injection of BAL in oil (10%) – systematic effects

Decontamination:
- Bleach
- Caustic soda

Notes:

Ethyldichloroarsine (ED)

Characteristics:
- Colorless to brown liquids.
- Soluble in most organic solvents but poorly in water.
- More volatile than mustard.
- Fruity, biting and irritating odor.
- As liquid penetrates rubber and most impermeable fabrics.
- Irritating effect on nose and throat – intolerable at 1 minute.
- Blistering less delayed than HD.
- Persistency - short

Toxicology:
- Median detectable concentration – nasal and throat irritation.
- Median Incapacitating dosage:
    - Inhalation – 5 to 10 mg-min/m^3
- Median Lethal dosage:
    - Inhalation – 3,000 to 5,000 mg-min/m^3
    - Skin absorption – 100,000 mg-min/m^3

ED

Physical Findings:

Organ/System	Symptomology
Skin	Erythema Thick roofed blisters Yellowish blister fluid - nontoxic
Eyes	Pain and blepharospasm occur instantly. Edema of conjunctivae and lids.
Pulmonary	Pulmonary edema
Systemic	Systemic poisoning Acute poisoning result in hypovolemic shock.

Protection Required:

- Protective mask
- Permeable protective clothing for vapor and small droplets.
- Impermeable clothing for large

droplets, splashes and smears.

Medical Management:
- BAL ointment – skin
- Morphine – pain
- Atropine sulfate ointment – eyes
- Intramuscular injection of BAL in oil (10%) – systematic effects.

Decontamination:
- Bleach
- Caustic soda

Notes:

ED

Phosgene (CG)

Characteristics:

- Odor of newly mown hay or freshly cut grass or corn.
- Colorless gas
- Extremely volatile
- Non-persistent but may remain for long periods of time in low-lying areas.
- Soluble in organic solvents and fatty oils.
- Rapidly hydrolyzed in water forming hydrochloric acid and carbon dioxide.

Toxicology:

- Phosgene irritates the mucous membranes at 4 mg/m^3
- Median Incapacitating dosage – 1,600 mg-min/m^3
- Median Lethal dosage – 3200 mg-min/m^3

Physical Findings:

Organ/System	Symptomology
Eyes	Lacrimation
Gastrointestinal	Nausea Vomiting
Pulmonary	Coughing Choking Chest tightness Rales and rhonchi Delayed pulmonary edema (4 hours from exposure). Hypoxia
Systemic	Hypotension

Protection Required:
- Protective mask or gas-particulate filter unit.
- Protection required – gas mask and PPE

Medical Management:
- Terminate exposure
- Execute ABCs

- Enforce rest – minimal physical exertion.
- Manage airway secretions and prevent treat bronchospasm.
- Antibiotics for infection
- Bronchodilators for bronchospasm
- Steroid therapy for bronchospasm and damaged airway.
- Prevent/treat pulmonary edema
- Positive airway pressure
- IV fluid administration
- Prevent/treat hypoxia
- Oxygen therapy
- Intubation/ventilation
- Prevent/treat hypotension
- IV administration of crystalloid or colloid.
- Vasopressors

Decontamination:
- Vapor – Fresh air
- Liquid – Irrigation with copious amounts of water.

Chlorine (CL)

Characteristics:
- Greenish-yellow liquefied gas.
- Pungent, irritating odor
- Reacts violently with ammonia, acetylene, ether, turpentine, hydrogen, and fuel gas.
- Dry chlorine noncorrosive at normal temperatures.
- Moist chlorine very corrosive.
- Heavier than air.
- Soluble in water.

Toxicology:
- Median Incapacitating dosage (unmasked) – 1,800 mg-min/m^3
- Median Lethal dosage – 19,000 mg-min/m^3

CL

Physical Findings:

Ingestion	Inhalation
Severe pain mouth	Weakness
Fever	Tight chest
Inability to breath due to throat swelling shut.	Feeling of suffocation.
Severe pain in throat.	Coughing
Severe abdominal pain.	Shortness of breath.
Vomit containing dark colored blood.	Coughing up blood.
Rapid drop in blood pressure.	Choking
	Cyanotic
	Low blood pressure
	Dizziness

Protection Required:

- Protective mask
- Protective clothing if working in chemical environment.

C-4-128

Medical Management:

Symptoms	Treatment
Eye pain	Irrigation with copious amount of water.
Gastrointestinal	Give fluids Give milk of magnesia Treat the symptoms
Pulmonary	Remove to fresh air Oxygen Intubation and ventilation

Decontamination:
- Large amounts of water.
- If chlorine on skin or in eyes, flush with water for 15 minutes.

Notes:

Hydrogen Cyanide (AC)

Characteristics:

- Odor of peach kernels or bitter almonds.
- Absorbed into the body primarily by breathing.
- Prevents normal utilization of oxygen.
- Colorless, highly volatile liquid
- Highly soluble and stable in water.
- In the gaseous state it dissipates quickly in the air.
- Very rapid action – death within 15 minutes after lethal dosage.

Toxicology:

- Incapacitating dosage – varies with concentration.
- Lethal dosage:
  - Concentration at 200 mg/m^3 – lethal dosage of 2,000 mg-min/m^3
  - Concentration at 150 mg/m^3 – lethal dosage of 4,500 mg-min/m^3

AC

Physical Findings:

Moderate Low Concentration of Vapor	Severe High Concentration of Vapor
Increase in rate and depth of breathing.	Increase in rate and depth of breathing - 15 seconds.
Dizziness	Convulsions - 30 seconds
Nausea	Cessation of respiration 2-4 minutes
Vomiting	Cessation of heartbeat 4-8 minutes
Headache	
Progress to severe with continued exposure.	

Protection Required:
- Protective mask
- Protective clothing when exposed or handling liquid AC.

AC

Medical Management:
- Antidote
- IV sodium nitrate
- IV sodium thisulfate
- Supportive therapy
- Oxygen
- Correct acidosis

Decontamination:
- Skin decontamination not usually necessary.
- Wet, contaminated clothing removed.
- Underlying skin decontaminated with water.

Notes:

Cyanogen Chloride (CK)

Characteristics:
- Odor unnoticed due to severe irritating and lacrimating properties.
- Absorbed into the body primarily by breathing.
- Prevents normal utilization of oxygen.
- Colorless, highly volatile liquid
- Slightly soluble in water
- Dissolves in organic solvents
- Non-persistent but CK vapor will remain in thick brush area.

Toxicology:
- Incapacitating dosage – 7,000 mg-min/m^3
- Lethal dosage – 11,000 mg-min/m^3

CK

Physical Findings:

Moderate Low Concentration of Vapor	Severe High Concentration of Vapor
Increase in rate and depth of breathing.	Increase in rate and depth of breathing - 15 seconds.
Dizziness	Convulsions - 30 seconds
Nausea	Cessation of respiration 2-4 minutes
Vomiting	Cessation of heartbeat 4-8 minutes
Headache	
Progress to severe with continued exposure.	

Protection Required:
- Protective mask
- Very high concentration may overpower mask filters.

C-5-134

Medical Management:
- Antidote
- IV sodium nitrate
- IV sodium thisulfate
- Supportive therapy
- Oxygen
- Correct acidosis

Decontamination:
- Skin decontamination not usually necessary.
- Wet, contaminated clothing removed.
- Underlying skin decontaminated with water.

Notes:

Arsine (SA)

Characteristics:
- Highest volatility of compounds to use as chemical agents.
- Ignites easily so can't be used with explosives.
- Mild garlic-like odor
- Primarily dispersed as vapor.
- Rate of action – 2 hours to 11 days
- Short persistency

Toxicology:
- Incapacitating dosage – 2,500 mg-min/m^3
- Lethal dosage – 5,000 mg-min/m^3

Physical Findings:

Slight Exposure	Increased Exposure	Severe Exposure
Headache	Chills	Damage to blood
Uneasiness	Nausea	Damages liver
	Vomiting	Damages kidneys
		Anemia

Protection Required:
• Protective mask

Medical Management:
• Symptomatic relief - administration of antiemetic such as trimethobenzamide hydrochloride IM, IV, orally, or rectally.
• Analgesic for headache.

Decontamination:
• None

SA

Adamsite (DM)

Characteristics:
- No pronounced odor.
- Very high rate of action – 1 minute required for temporary incapacitation at concentration of $22mg/m^3$.
- Disseminated as an aerosol.
- Persistency is short.

Toxicology:
- Incapacitating dosage
- 22 mg-min/m^3 – 1 minute exposure
- 8 mg-min/m^3 – 60 minutes exposure
- Lethal dosage – $15,000$ mg-min/m^3

Physical Findings (progressive order):
- Irritation of the eyes and mucous membranes.
- Viscous discharge from the nose similar to cold.
- Sneezing and coughing

- Severe headache
- Acute pain and tightness in chest.
- Nausea
- Vomiting
- Moderate concentrations – effects last 30 minutes
- High concentrations – effects may last 3 3hours

Protection Required:
- Protective mask

Medical Management:
- Symptomatic relief – administration of antiemetic such as trimethobenzamide hydrochloride IM, IV, orally, or rectally.
- Analgesic for headache

Decontamination:
- None needed in open area.
- Bleaching powder for gross contamination in enclosed places.

Notes:

SECTION D

<u>Decontamination</u>

D-1 - Introduction

D-2 - Establishing Decon Zone.

D-3 - Decon Methods and Solutions.

D-4 - Decon of Personnel/Walking Wounded, Non-Ambulatory Patients, and Mass Decon.

D-5 - Equipment Decon

Introduction:

Decontamination is the process of reducing and preventing the spread of contamination from persons (victims) and equipment at a CB event through the use of physical or chemical means. First Responders and Incident Commanders (ICs) should implement a technically sound and thorough decontamination process until the incident has been mitigated and the need for decon is no longer necessary.

The primary object of decontamination is to avoid becoming contaminated or contaminating other person(s) or equipment outside of an established HOT ZONE.

Decontamination Considerations:
(DHHS/PHS ATSDR Managing Hazardous Materials Incidents)

Wind Direction

The direction of the wind is very important during decon. Patient decontamination should take place upwind and away from the patient arrival area. A decon site should initially be set up to take advantage of a prevailing wind. Plans should be incorporated for quick rearrangement if the direction of the wind changes more than 45 degrees. ICs should wait for 15-20 minutes to determine if wind conditions require further change before a move. If a change is made the site needs to be moved at least 75 meters upwind. Personnel working in the old "clean" area when the wind shifts must make sure that all casualties remain masked. The unforeseeable changing of winds illustrates that ideally the decon setup should include two separate (planned) decon sites about 75 meters apart.

Decon Site Security:
Security at the decon site should be strongly enforced to prevent unsuspecting individuals from spreading contamination to and from the area. Security provisions should also take into consideration the potential risk of further attacks and media convergence.

Control of Decon Site:
The control of personnel and victim movement is necessary to ensure that further contamination is avoided at all cost. The hot line must be secured and enforced.

Decon Site Logistics:
Provisions must be made to ensure that decon and medical personnel are supplied and equipped to manage and decon contaminated casualties.

Hotline:
A hotline is an arbitrary line that separates the area of agent contamination from one

that is agent free. Once the hot line has been established it should be clearly marked using yellow caution tape or other markers to ensure that person(s) with potential contamination do not cross into a clean area. The only entrance to the clean treatment area is through decontamination stations.

Notes:

The area between the hot zone and the support zone is the decon zone. It should be established near the incident area. The following factors should be considered when determining the decon zone:

- Upwind, and uphill from the hot zone.
- The natural ventilation of the atmosphere will allow for dispersal of vapor gassing-off from contaminated victims.
- Located in areas where adequate supplies and electricity are or can be made available.
- An additional area close by which can resupply the necessary supplies to personnel working in the decon area.

Decontamination Station:

A decon station (see fig. 1) must have the ability to be staffed rapidly either prior to an incident or immediately after notification of a CB event. A station must have the ability to perform decontamination concurrently with life saving measures for people suffering from agent exposure or other injuries.

A decontamination station should provide:
- Overhead protection such as plastic sheeting, trailer covers, ponchos, etc.
- Procedures for handling of property.
- Be able to collect and contain all used decon solutions and rinse water for later disposition.
- A station should have procedures for dealing with infants, handicapped persons, and the elderly who are also likely to be exposed during a release.
- Consider the fact that the police or others with an interest will want to be in the decon area to collect evidence and interview victims.

The staff assigned to a decon station should be able to decon a minimum number of victims prior to establishing a working station. During the placement and setup phase of the station a decon team should begin a screening process of victims in order to determine the potential number to be decontaminated.

Two decon areas may be established when dealing with two large active incidents. One for litter casualties and one for walking wounded. Both stations should be designed, equipped and staffed to provide a sequence of decontamination functions for contaminated individuals. With minimal assistance from attendants (other than directions), most victims should be able to proceed through the decon sequence on their own. Those who are injured or handicapped, however, may require the assistance of attendants or special equipment (stretcher, wheelchair etc.). People requiring extensive handling should be considered a litter patient in-order to expedite the process. A location about 75 meters from the working decon area is needed for each decon station. The area is to allow workers to rehabilitate and remove masks and equipment. Without a clean rest area, workers must remain in protective gear even during rest.

Figure 1

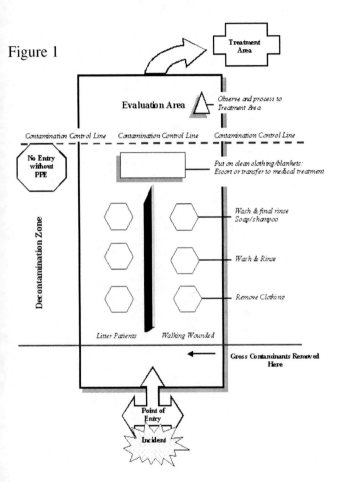

Treatment Area

Evaluation Area — Observe and process to Treatment Area

Contamination Control Line   Contamination Control Line   Contamination Control Line

No Entry without PPE

Put on clean clothing/blankets: Escort or transfer to medical treatment

Decontamination Zone

Wash & final rinse Soap/shampoo

Wash & Rinse

Remove Clothing

Litter Patients   Walking Wounded

Gross Contaminants Removed Here

Point of Entry

Incident

D-2-149

Figure 2

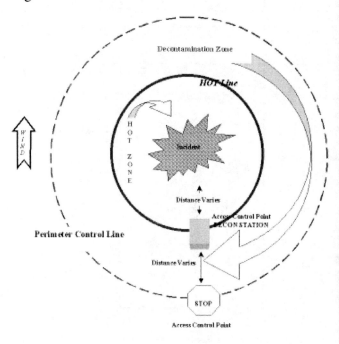

Decontamination Zone

HOT Line

WIND

HOT ZONE

Incident

Distance Varies

Access Control Point
DECON STATION

Perimeter Control Line

Distance Varies

STOP

Access Control Point

D-3 - Decon Methods and Solutions

(NFPA 471 - Recommended for Practice for Responding to Hazardous Materials Incidents, 1997 Edition)

The two basic methods of decontamination first responders should be familiar with are the physical removal, and chemical removal (deactivation) of agents.

Physical Methods:
Physical methods of decontamination generally involve the physical removal of the contaminant from the contaminated person or object along with containment of the contaminant for appropriate disposal.

Examples of physical decontamination include:
- Absorption
- Brushing and scrapping
- Isolation and disposal
- Vacuuming
- Washing

The scraping of an area with a wooden stick, i.e., a tongue depressor or stick, can remove bulk agent by physical means. The overall benefit to most physical removal methods is their generic applications. All physical removal methods work equally well on chemical agents regardless of the chemical composition. Knowledge of the specific contaminating agent or agents is not needed.

Chemical Methods:
The use of chemical decontamination methods are primarily used on equipment and surfaces and not on people (victims). The chemical decontamination method generally involves the use of some type of chemical reaction in an effort to render the contaminant less harmful to the object and environment. In some cases of etiological contaminants, chemical methods are actually biologically "killing" the organism.

Examples of chemical methods include the following:
  • Absorption

- Chemical degradation
- Disinfecting or sterilization
- Neutralization
- Solidification

Some decontamination studies have been done testing the effectiveness of common household products in decontamination procedures. The rapid use of water, soap and water, and flour followed by wet tissue wipes produced results equal, or in some instances better than those produced by the use of Fuller's Earth, Dutch Powder, and other compounds. ***However, more important than the method used, is how and when it is used.***

Absorbent Materials:
Using adsorbent material as a decontaminate is an effective way to reduce the quantity of chemical agent available for intake through the skin. In emergency situations dry powders such as soap detergents, earth, and flour, may be useful. Flour followed by

wiping with wet tissue paper has been effective against GD, VX and HD.

Water/Soap Wash:
Water and water/soap solutions can physically remove or dilute agents. In the absence of Hypochlorite solutions or other decon methods, the use of these methods are considered reasonable options. Fresh water and seawater can remove chemical agents through stream force from a fire hose and via slow hydrolysis.

Flushing with Water or Aqueous Solutions:
Copious flushing with water can physically remove an agent. The use of fire department hoses and a spray nozzle can achieve this. However, considerations need to be made for wastewater and water temperature. Wastewater needs to be collected and water temperature could cause hypothermia in some victims and personnel.

Hypo-chlorite Solutions:

Two different types or "concentrations" of chlorine solution can be used in personnel and victim decon. A 0.5% chlorine solution is the primary solution for all patient washing procedures. It is described in detailed in the decon procedure section D-3. A 5% chlorine solution is used for the decon of equipment e.g., scissors, aprons and gloves that are used by personnel working within the patient decon area.

Both types of hypo-chlorite solutions may be made using 6-ounces Calcium hypo-chlorite (HTH). The 0.5% solution can be made adding one six ounce container of calcium hypo-chlorite to five gallons of water.

By adding eight, six-ounce containers of calcium hypo-chlorite to five gallons of water, you can make the 5% solution. The solutions should be made up fresh with a pH in the alkaline range. Once prepared they should be placed in buckets for use in the decon area. The buckets should be distinctly marked for purposes of identification between the 5% chlorine solution and the 0.5% solutions.

Notes:

(EMS Safety Techniques & Applications, USFA Publication, 1994)

As a First Responder, you may become exposed to a CB agent during an incident. It is vital that you do not panic if you suspect you have been exposed. Prevention of further exposure and survival depends on the steps you take immediately to physically remove the agent. The self or buddy decon method will be useful to personnel and walking wounded because of its relative ease. When adequate resources are available, contaminated personnel and walking wounded should be entered into separated male and female stations.

SELF/BUDDY/WALKING WOUNDED DECONTAMINATION

Step 1:
Remove signs of gross contamination by scraping, sweeping or blotting the material away.

Step 2:
Remove clothing or equipment rapidly but cautiously. Clothing should be pulled away from the body. In the event clothing needs to be removed over the head, cut it away.

Step 3:
Wash hands prior to continuing the process.

Step 4:
Remove all external extraneous items from contact with the body. Such items include hearing aids, watches, toupees, artificial limbs. (Note: If the victim or rescuer cannot safely evacuate the area without eyeglasses they should be allowed to sit in a Hypochlorite solution for at least five minutes.)

Step 5:
After removing eyeglasses or contact lenses flush the eyes with large amounts of water.

Step 6:
Gently wash face and hair with soap and lukewarm water, followed by a thorough rinse with lukewarm water.

Step 7:
Begin to decon other body surfaces starting from the neck down using a supplied solution blot (not swabbing or wiping) with a cloth. Wash the same areas in lukewarm soapy water and rinse in clear lukewarm water. In the absence of a Hypochlorite solution, copious amounts of lukewarm soapy water and rinsing with lukewarm water is useful.

Step 8:
Change into uncontaminated clothing or blankets and await further instructions.

NON-AMBULATORY DECONTAMINATION PROCESS

If victims are unconscious, seriously injured, or require extra care during the process, treat them as litter patients. The only real difference for the decon process for litter patients is that more personnel and resources are required. The following procedure is necessary to decontaminate a litter patient. Walking wounded can also be incorporated into this process.

Step 1:
Remove signs of gross contamination from the victim prior to entering decon station.

Step 2:
Transfer patient to a decon preparation litter and cut away all clothing. Remove all personal property and then transfer the patient to a decontamination litter or a canvas litter with a plastic sheeting cover. All property should be bagged, secured, clearly identified. A copy of the tag should be placed with the victim for control purposes.

Step 3:
Eyeglasses and contacts should be removed.
- Rescuers will decon hands by blotting with solution then thoroughly rinsing with water before removing contact lenses. A contact lens remover should be used to decrease the risk of cross contamination.
- Contact lens should be collected and disposed of.
- Eyeglasses in metal frames can be deconed in a five-minute bath of solution followed by through rinsing.
- If eyeglass are in a composite or plastic frame they should be secured in an impermeable bag for later decon.

Step 4:
Decon team members decon their gloves and aprons with the 5% Hypochlorite solution.

Step 5:
Victim's skin should be blotted with the solution excluding the face. Superficial wounds are flushed with a 0.5% Hypochlo-

rite solution and new dressings applied as needed. Splints are not removed but saturated to the skin with 0.5% solution. If the splint cannot be saturated, it must be removed sufficiently so that everything below the splint can be saturated with the 0.5% Hypochlorite solution.

Step 6:
Place victim into a shower and flush with copious amounts of water. Start with the face and hands.

Step 7:
Check the victim for signs of contamination and carry out medical screening procedures.

Step 8:
Following successful decon, transport the victim to the support area for clothing and evaluation and observation.

Step 9:
Each individual should be marked and identified as such. This can be accomplished

with a tag, triage tag, or writing on a victims forehead.

During processing each victim should receive a certificate indicating:
- Description of decon actions taken.
- Time decon complete.
- Release form from observation area.
- Any medical treatment performed in conjunction with decon.
- A copy should also go to decon record management.

Final Monitoring:

Monitor victims for possible further contamination using a chemical agent monitor or other methods available. Once a victim is confirmed "clean" of a chemical agent, he or she can be transferred via a shuffle pit over the contamination control line.

A shuffle pit consists of two parts super tropical bleach (STB) and three parts earth or sand. The pit should be deep enough to

cover the bottom of the protective over-
boots. A washing of the decon apron and
gloves in 5.0% Hypo-chlorite solution pre-
cedes the transfer of the victim to a new
clean stretcher. The victim can then proceed
to the next station.

MASS DECONTAMINATION:
When confronted with large amounts of
victim(s) requiring decontamination the
previously recommended decon procedures
must be followed. It is imperative that all
personnel and victim(s) are decontaminated
to prevent further or cross-contamination.

In order to gain some means of control of a
large crowd, which is contaminated:
- Communicate with them via a PA or
loud speaker.
- Tell them to try and remain calm and
that help is on the way.
- Try to categorize the ambulatory and
non-ambulatory victims into to
distinctive decon lines.
- Provide ample protection for the Site

and Triage Recon Team.
• You will have to establish a priority for the victims in order to facilitate an effective decontamination and treatment procedure.
• Continue to COMMUNICATE with the crowd.
• If it is impossible to establish a HOT ZONE, utilize a fire hose to begin decon and keep the crowd back.

Notes:

D-5 - Equipment Decon

(DHHS/PHS ATSDR Managing Hazardous Materials Incidents; Hazardous Materials Exposure Emergency Response and Patient Care, Brady Book, 1991)

Nylon and canvas equipment bags can be decontaminated by boiling them for one hour in water. Soap in the water will speed-up the process. After removal from the boiling water, rinse, air-dry, and return the items to service. This kind of equipment can also be decontaminated with bleach slurry methods as well.

Leather equipment like gun belts can quickly absorb liquid chemical agents. Initial decon should be done as rapidly as possible. For a thorough decon, soak shoes, straps, and other leather equipment in water heated to 122°F to 131°F (50°C to 55°C) for 4-6 hours, then air dry without excess heat.

Liquid contaminants on impermeable protective clothing (Impermeable Protective

Clothing, Aprons, Gloves, and Boots) should be neutralized or removed. The quickest decon method (physical removal) can be performed while clothing is still on. If slurries are not available, blot liquid off with available material (for example, rags). This should be done immediately if splashes or large drops of agent are on clothing. A complete decon, however, can be accomplished by one of the following methods:

Aeration:
If the contamination is light or is caused by vapor, articles can be decontaminated by airing outdoors for several days.

Water:
Immerse heavily contaminated articles in hot soapy water at a temperature just below boiling for 1 hour. Do not stir or agitate. After 1 hour, remove the articles, rinse in clear water, and drain. While items are still hot and wet, pull apart any surfaces that are stuck together. Hang them up to dry. Repeat the process if necessary.

Slurry:

Decontaminate impregnated items (worn by personnel) by spraying or applying slurry immediately after contamination. After a few minutes, wash off the slurry with water. This can be done while the clothing is on.

Decontamination of Stretchers:

To provide emergency protection for canvas or metal stretchers, cover them with materials such as ponchos, or plastic sheeting. Depending upon what type of patient stretcher was used during an incident, all of them must be properly decontaminated to prevent further hazard of exposure.

Canvas Litter:

Decontaminate canvas by immersion in boiling water for 1 hour. If available, add 4 pounds of sodium carbonate (washing soda) to each 10 gallons of water. After boiling with washing soda, rinse with clear water.

Wood Litter:

Apply 30% aqueous slurry of bleach and let it react for 12-24 hours. Repeat applications if necessary, then swab the wood dry and let it aerate at elevated temperatures, if possible.

Metal Stretcher and Wheelchair:

If the litter/wheelchair cannot be taken apart, decontaminate it with bleach slurry or by flushing it with hot soapy water. It is effective for all chemical agents. Apply this solution to all contaminated surfaces by spray, broom, or swab; after 30 minutes, flush with water. After decon, aerate the metal outdoors for several hours. (If wheels of the wheelchair cannot be effectively decontaminated, they must be destroyed.)

Notes:

Reference

E-1 - Chem-Bio Methods of Delivery

E-2 - Precursors - Dual-Use Chemicals

E-3 - START Triage System

Introduction:

The methods which a terrorist or attacker could use to deploy CB weapons are essentially the same for both weapons with the exception of indirect transmission of a biological agent through infection.

In a CB attack it has been said that "The smaller the target, the more likely the terrorists are to succeed, especially if the target population resides or works within a closed area."

Methods:

CB dissemination devices used in the past have typically been simple in design and operation. However, in 13% of the total cases, the dissemination was by an "unknown" delivery method. Listed below are a total of eight known dissemination techniques that have been used in past CB incidents:

- Contamination of food or drink (43%)

- Contamination of consumable products (13%).
- Contamination of water supplies (12%).
- Aerosols (9%)
- Contaminated personal items (e.g., clothing) (4%)
- Contaminated projectiles (3%)
- Disease vectors (2%)
- Vapor clouds (1%).

In planning an attack, a terrorist or criminal most choose the delivery system carefully. The terrorist or attacker must in all cases have:

- Prior knowledge of the spaces, size, airflow, and layout.
- A precise knowledge of the physical properties of the CB agent being used.

Chemical Agents:
Generally speaking, a chemical weapon is comprised of two parts:

- The chemical agent.
- The means of delivering it.

Chemical agents are extremely deadly in

large and small quantities. Optimally, the delivery system should disseminate the agent – most often a liquid – as a cloud of droplets, known as an aerosol.

The most effective way for a terrorist to execute a "mass" chemical attack is to disseminate a chemical agent in an enclosed space such as a hotel, office building, school, or convention center with a resulting casualty toll ranging between a few hundred and several thousand.

Biological Agents:
BW agents are nonvolatile solids that are best disseminated as liquid slurry or a dry powder of freeze-dried organisms or toxin. BW agents are far more toxic than CW agents and pound for pound can cover a wider area than CW.

BW delivery systems can range in complexity and effectiveness from an agricultural sprayer, mounted on a vehicle to a remotely activated room freshener device. The key in effective delivery of a BW agent is the generation of an aerosol or stable cloud of suspended microscopic droplets, each containing from one to thousands of bacteria or virus. A fog or a smoke is an example of visible aerosols.

CB Methods of Delivery
The following are some of the methods that a terrorist could use to disseminate a CB agent.

Spray Devices
• Through the use of commercial spray-ing equipment (i.e. with a paint sprayer or insecticide sprayer a terrorist could attack a crowd quickly and effectively.)

• An attack on a stadium full of fans using a low-flying crop-duster-type aircraft (helicopter, single engine banner towing aircraft, RC blimp) might kill thousands.

• A hand-held liquid spray gun similar to a tear gas dispenser might appeal to terror-ists willing to confront victims directly.

• Or a suicide squad armed with multiple

devices could create an enormous number of casualties in crowded areas such as airport terminals or shopping malls.

• The covert placement of a remotely activated sprayer in an enclosed space (HVAC) could kill all in the area or building with little or no warning of the attack.

Explosive/Bursting Devices
Although dispersion by explosive means usually results in a significant loss of agent on detonation. The primary objective of this method is to either scatter the agent in the air creating a vapor cloud, or to heavily contaminate the immediate or surrounding area. Explosive dissemination often results in a mix of both effects. While not as efficient as a spray device, explosive dissemination is a simple and reliable approach.

• Properly placed chemical bombs could be exploded in a crowded area (stadium, airport) injuring or killing hundreds.

• A truck loaded with drums or canisters containing a nerve agent like VX or Sarin could be crashed into a building and exploded, turning the deadly substance into a fine mist that would envelop the entire facility.

- Chemical agents could also be used effectively as contaminants for projectiles such as bullets, flechettes, and shrapnel.

Breaking Devices

Breaking devices are devices that encapsulate a CB agent and release it when it is broken. They can be constructed from common items (light bulb, thermos bottles).

Contamination (dumping/placing)

Contrary to popular belief, the water supply is not a highly vulnerable target. Generally the bulk of water drawn from an urban water supply never comes into physical contact with the population; it waters lawns, washes clothes, flushes toilets, cools industrial equipment, etc. Any of the highly lethal biological agents are not effectively transmitted by water and would be further debilitated by hydrolysis, chlorination, and purification systems.

The contamination of a municipal water supply would require compensation for a significant dilution factor and hence quantities of CB agent which are beyond what terrorists or attackers might find easy to acquire or produce.

Contamination of foodstuffs is one likely avenue for the terrorist. CB Agents could be inserted into production lines at factories turning out packaged prepared foods, the same foods that come in 'tamper-proof' containers. Also, attacks through bulk foodstuffs or beverages (via dairies, meat processing plants, and soda and beer bottlers) are another possibility.

Vectors (Biological)
A vector is the carrier of the bacteria, and could be an insect, rodent, or human. A vector could also be an item such as clothing, water, or food.

Production of chemical agents is typically a multi-phase endeavor requiring several chemical precursors. Many of these chemicals have numerous legitimate purposes in industry. However, when discovered outside of their typical setting, they serve as excellent indicators of agent production. Foreknowledge of what chemicals have direct relevance to chemical agent production enables responders to recognize activities potentially directed toward the creation of chemical agent. The following table lists chemical agent precursor chemicals and links them to their related agent and their civil uses.

Precursor Chemical	Units of agent per-unit of precursor	CW Agent Production	Civil Uses
Thiodiglycol 111-48-8	1.3	Sulfur Mustard - HD	Organic Synthesis Carrier for dyes in textile industry Lubricant additives Manufacturing of plastics
Phosphorous oxychloride 10025-87-3	1.05	Tabun - GA	Organic Synthesis Plasticizers Gasoline Additives Hydraulic Fluids Insecticides Flame retardants
Dimethyl methylphosphonate (DMMP) 756-79-6	1.12 1.45	Sarin GB Soman GD GF	Flame Retardants

Precursor Chemical	Units of agent per-unit of precursor	CW Agent Production	Civil Uses
Methylphosphonate difluoride 676-99-3	1.40 1.82 1.80	Sarin GB Soman GD GF	Organic Synthesis Specific uses not identified.
Methylphophonyl dichloride 676-97-1	1.05 1.36 1.35	Sarin GB Soman GD GF	Organic Synthesis Specific uses not identified.
Dimethylphosphite 868-85-9	1.27 1.65 1.65	Sarin GB Soman GD GF	Organic Synthesis Lubricant Additive

Precursor Chemical	Units of agent per-unit of precursor	CW Agent Production	Civil Uses
Phosphorus trichloride 7719-12-2	1.95 1.18 1.02	VG Tabun (GA) Sarin (GB) *Salt Process*	Organic Synthesis Insecticides Gasoline Additives Plasticizers
	1.32	Soman (GD) *Salt Process*	Surfactants
	1.31	GF *Salt Process*	Dyestuff

Precursor Chemical	Units of agent per-unit of precursor	CW Agent Production	Civil Uses
Thionyl chloride[2] 7719-09-7	1.18 1.53 1.51 1.34 0.714 0.655 1.145	Sarin (GB) Soman (GD) GF Sulfur Mustard (HD) Nitrogen Mustard HN1 Nitrogen Mustard HN2 Nitrogen Mustard HN3	Organic Synthesis Catalyst Pesticide Engineering Plastics
2-Chloro-N,N-diisopropylethylamine 96-79-7	1.64 1.72	VX VS	Organic Synthesis

Precursor Chemical	Units of agent per-unit of precursor	CW Agent Production	Civil Uses
Diisopropylaminoethan-ethiol 5842-07-9	1.66 1.75	VX VS	Organic Synthesis
Potassium Fluoride 7789-28-3	2.41 3.14 3.10	Sarin (GB) Soman (GD) GF	Fluorination of organic compounds. Cleaning disinfecting of brewery, dairy, and other food processing equipment. Glass and Porcelain equipment
2-Chloroethanol 107-07-3	0.99 1.06	Sulfur Mustard (HD) Nitrogen Mustard (HN1)	Organic Synthesis Insecticides Solvent

Precursor Chemical	Units of agent per-unit of precursor	CW Agent Production	Civil Uses
Dimethylamine 124-40-3	3.61	Tabun (GA)	Organic Synthesis Pharmaceuticals Detergents Pesticides Gasoline Additives Missile Fuels Vulcanization of rubber.
Diethyl ethylphosphonate 78-38-6	0.93	Eythl Sarin (GE)	Heavy Metal Extraction
Diethyl N,N-dimethyl phosphoramidate 2404-03-7	0.90	Tabun (GA)	Organic Synthesis Specific uses not identified.

Precursor Chemical	Units of agent per-unit of precursor	CW Agent Production	Civil Uses
Diethyl phosphite 762-04-9	1.02 1.32 1.30	Sarin (GB) Soman (GD) GF	Paint Solvent Lubricant Additive
Dimethylamine HCl 506-59-2	1.99	Tabun (GA)	Organic Synthesis Pharmaceuticals Surfactants Pesticides Gasoline Additives
Hydrogen fluoride 7664-39-3	7.0 9.11 9.01	Sarin (GB) Soman (GD) GF	Fluorinating agent in chemical reactions. Catalyst in alkylation and polymerization reactions. Uranium refining

Precursor Chemical	Units of agent per-unit of precursor	CW Agent Production	Civil Uses
Methyl benzilate 76-89-1	1.39	BZ	Organic Synthesis Tranquilizers
Methylphosphonous dichloride 676-83-5	2.28	VX	Organic Synthesis
N,N-Diisopropyl-2-aminoethanol 96-80-0	1.84	VX	Organic Synthesis Specific uses not identified.
Pinacolyl alcohol 464-07-3	1.79	Soman (GD)	Specific uses not identified.

Precursor Chemical	Units of agent per-unit of precursor	CW Agent Production	Civil Uses
O-ethyl.2-diisopopyl aminoethyl methylphosphonate (QL) 57856-11-8	1.14	VX	Specific uses not identified.
Arsenic trichloride 7784-34-1	0.43 1.14 1.53	Arsine Lewisite Adamsite (DM)	Organic Synthesis Pharmaceuticals Insecticides Ceramics
Benzilic Acid 76-93-7	1.48	BZ	Organic Synthesis
Diethyl methylphosphonite 15715-41-0	1.97	VX	Organic Synthesis

Precursor Chemical	Units of agent per-unit of precursor	CW Agent Production	Civil Uses
Dimethyl ethylphosphonate 6163-75-3	1.12	Ethyl Sarin (GE)	Organic Synthesis
Ethylphosphonous difluoride 430-78-4	1.57	Ethyl Sarin (GE)	Organic Synthesis
Methylphosphonous difluoride 753-59-3	3.16 1.67 2.17 2.15	VX Sarin (GB) Soman (GD) GF	Organic Synthesis
3-Quinuclidone 1619-34-7	2.65	BZ	Hypotensive Agent Used in synthesis of pharmecuticals.

Precursor Chemical	Units of agent per-unit of precursor	CW Agent Production	Civil Uses
Phosphorous pentachloride 10026-13-8	0.78	Tabun (GA)	Organic Synthesis Pesticides Plastics
Pinacolone 75-97-8	1.82	Soman (GD)	Specific uses not identified.
Potassium Cyanide 151-50-8	1.25 0.41	Tabun (GA) Hydrogen cyanide	Extraction of gold and silver from ore. Pesticides Fumigants Electroplating

Precursor Chemical	Units of agent per-unit of precursor	CW Agent Production	Civil Uses
Sodium bifluoride 1333-83-1	2.26 2.94 2.91	Sarin (GB) Soman (GD) GF	Antiseptic Neutralizer in laundry operations. Tin plate production.
Sodium cyanide 143-33-9	1.65 0.55 1.25	Tabun (GA) Hydrogen Cyanide Cyanogen chloride	Gold & silver ore extraction. Fumigant Dye and pigment production. Metal core hardening Nylon production
Triethanolamine 102-71-6	1.37	Nitrogen Mustard HN3	Organic Synthesis Detergents Cosmetics Corrosion inhibitor Plasticizers Rubber accelerator

Precursor Chemical	Units of agent per-unit of precursor	CW Agent Production	Civil Uses
Phosphorus pentasulfide 1314-80-3	1.20	VX	Organic Synthesis Insecticides Mitocides Lubricant additives Pyrotechnics
Diisopropylamine 108-18-9	3.65	VX	Organic Synthesis Specific uses not identified.
Sodium sulfide 1313-82-2	2.04	Sulfur Mustard HD	Paper manufacturing Rubber manufacturing Metal refining Dye manufacturing

Precursor Chemical	Units of agent per-unit of precursor	CW Agent Production	Civil Uses
Sulfur monochloride (sulfur chloride) 10025-67-9	1.18	Sulfur Mustard HD	Organic Synthesis Pharmecuticals Sulfur dyes Insecticides Rubber vulcanization Polymerization catalyst Hardening of soft woods. Extraction of gold from ores.
Sulfur dichloride 10545-99-0	1.54	Sulfur Mustard HD	Organic Synthesis Rubber vulcanization Insecticides Vulcanizing Oils Chlorinating agent

Precursor Chemical	Units of agent per-unit of precursor	CW Agent Production	Civil Uses
Triethanolamine hydrochloride 637-39-8	1.10	Nitrogen Mustard	Organic Synthesis, Insecticides Surface active agents Waxes, polishes Textile specialties Lubricants, Toiletries Cement additives Petroleum demulsifier Synthetic resin
N.N-diisopropyl-2-aminoethyl chloride 96-79-7	1.34	VX	Organic Synthesis
Triethanolamine 102-71-6	1.37	Nitrogen Mustard HN3	Organic Synthesis Detergents, Cosmetics Corrosion inhibitor Plasticizer, Rubber accelerator

Introduction

The Simple Triage and Rapid Treatment (START) system is a simple and effective procedure, which allows first responders to triage patients at a MCI in one-minute or less.

The START system is based on three distinct observations made by a responder.

1. Respiration
2. Circulation
3. Mental Status

Research has determined that most trauma patients will die within the first hour [Golden Hour] after sustaining their injuries, mostly due to respiratory complications, excessive blood loss or head injury.

The Goal of Triage:
The Greatest Good for the Greatest Number!

FOUR START CATEGORIES

DECEASED Black Tag	No spontaneous effective respiration's present after an attempt to reposition the airway.
IMMEDIATE Red Tag	Respiration's present only after repositioning the airway. Applies to patients with respiratory rate >30. Capillary refill delayed more than 2 seconds. The patient fails to follow simple commands.
DELAYED Yellow Tag	Any patient who does not fit into the IMMEDIATE category or MINOR category.
MINOR Green Tag	Walking Wounded

How START Works

The rescuer or rescue team, which is assigned to triage victims, must place the victim's injuries into one of four categories.

START Procedure:
Respirations
Patients can be quickly assessed for respiratory rate and adequacy. If a patient is not breathing, check for foreign objects in the airway (dirt, dentures, and teeth). Reposition the head, using cervical spine precautions, if this does not delay the assessment.

If the above actions do not result in spontaneous respiration's, TAG the patient BLACK. If the patients respiration rate is greater than thirty per minute, TAG the patient RED. Patients with reparations of less than 30 per minute are not tagged at this time.

Perfusion
The best indicator for adequate perfusion is an assessment of capillary refill on the nailbed. Press a nailbed on a finger or lips and release. Capillary color should return to that area within 2 seconds. If it takes more

than 2 seconds, the patient is displaying signs of inadequate perfussion. TAG the patient RED. If the color does return within 2 seconds or less, the patient is not tagged until the next category.

If a patient's capillary refill cannot be assessed do to trauma to extremities or face, palpate the radial pulse. In most cases, if the radial pulse cannot be felt, the patient's systolic blood pressure is below 80mm Hg.

Hemorrhage control techniques will be incorporated into the next category. However, you can control significant bleeding by applying direct pressure and elevating the wounded extremity if necessary.

* Note utilize the "walking wounded" to assist in hemorrhage control on themselves or other patients when appropriate.

Mental Status

The evaluation of the patient's mental status is performed on patients whose respirations and perfusion are adequate and assessed in previous steps. The means which rescuers should use to test the mental status is ask the patient to:

- Open and close your eyes.
- Squeeze my hands.

If the patient cannot follow these commands, TAG the patient RED. If the patient can follow these commands, TAG the patient YELLOW.

Only after all the patients have been triaged using START can medical treatment begin. By effectively and efficiently using the START system, the above techniques should take no more than 60 seconds per patient. This means that a 2 man unit first on scene should be able to effectively triage 20 patients in 20 minutes if done properly.

CB Emergency Numbers
CHEMTREC
1-800-424-9300

US Public Health Service
1-800-872-6367

US Army Operations Center
1-800-851-8061

Domestic Preparedness Information Line
1-800-368-6498

National Response Center
1-800-424-8802